Sheldon S. Zinberg, M.D.

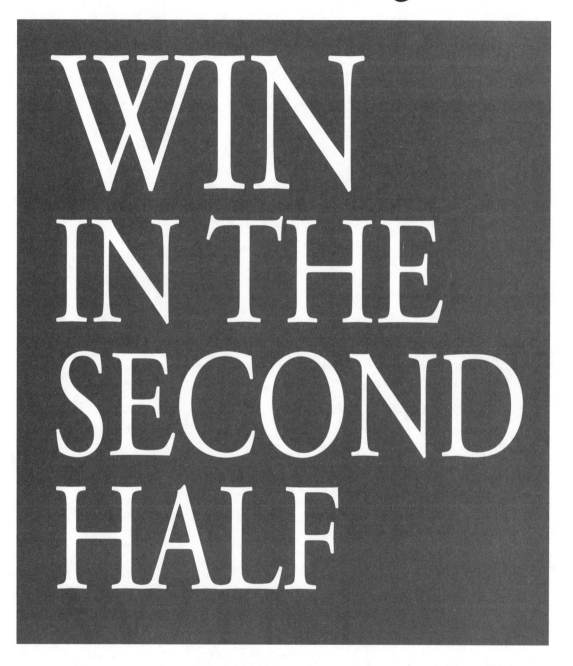

WIN IN THE SECOND HALF

A Guide to BETTER Aging and Fitness
for Men and Women

DEDICATION

This book is dedicated to all those that read it and implement the changes required to Win In the Second Half.

Illustrations by Melissa Huntington

SADDLEBACK PUBLISHING, INC.
Three Watson
Irvine, CA 92618-2767

E-MAIL: info@sdlback.com
Website: www.sdlback.com

ISBN 1 - 56254 - 074 - 2

Printed in the United States of America.

There are many people who played a role in making this book a reality. In part, it began as a family affair. The initial inspiration was derived from my son, Abram. He became genuinely exasperated by my unending and frequently explosive expressions of frustration in regard to the abundance of misinformation given to the public on the subjects of aging and fitness. He said, "Enough is enough, already. If it bothers you so much, write a book that separates the facts from the myths." And so I did. My wife, Nancy, was an indispensable asset as a research assistant and as an ex-officio editor. More importantly, the book could not have been completed without her encouragement and her gracious tolerance of my peculiar hours of toil. My daughter, Perri, has a doctorate in psychology. Her opinions and input on the sections dealing with sexual behavior in the mature adult, dementia, and mental exercise were enormously helpful.

Thomas Milano, Thomas Hatch, and their respective staffs skillfully formatted and edited the manuscript to make it more readable. Their patience and compassionately imposed discipline, in contending with my insatiable and seemingly infinite need to add and rewrite various sections, were essential to the completion of this volume. Melissa Huntington studied the manuscript and helped to clarify and enrich it with her artful and imaginative illustrations. The thousands of health experts, research scientists, and authors who have previously written on these subjects furnished a fount of information from which well-founded opinions could be formulated and articulated.

Last but most assuredly not least, I wish to thank all of my colleagues, friends, and patients for their invaluable opinions and ideas. Most deeply, I wish to thank my patients, the living and the deceased. The nature of their problems and how we dealt with them together was the most inspiring impetus for this writing.

CHAPTER THREE

Our Mental Muscle   35

Plaques and tangles,

Tangles and plaques,

Our mind it mangles,

And some it cracks.

CHAPTER FOUR

Brainaerobics and Mindercises   49

Your mind is your mate;

You govern its state.

You open its gate,

When you concentrate.

CHAPTER FIVE

Your Magic Bullet 59

Learn the stuff

That soon will follow,

And forget the guff

That others swallow.

CHAPTER SIX

Groans, Grumbles, and Gases 75

Breathe clean air,

Eat good greens,

If you care –

Here's the means.

CHAPTER SEVEN

Fiber, Vitamins, and Herbs   *93*

Now the saga shall begin

About your favorite vitamin.

Is what you know about your herb

A "not so scientific" blurb?

CHAPTER EIGHT

Minerals, Hormones,
Skin, and Bones   117

Try your best

To tie the suture

That makes your nest

A better future.

CHAPTER NINE

About Exercise   139

On a pound of fat,

Let me make my case—

A pound of muscle,

Takes less space.

CHAPTER TEN

Stretching   159

Prevent contractures,

Prevent that sprain,

Prevent those fractures,

And hold the gain.

CHAPTER ELEVEN

Strength Training   175

More muscle will build

From the sweat you have spilled.

So please try to continue

To bring forth what's in you.

CHAPTER TWELVE

Strength and Balance Exercises You Can Do at Home   199

Your balance is improved

And your agility grooved,

If you just take a seat

And repeat and repeat.

CHAPTER THIRTEEN

*Aerobic Exercise and Maintaining
Your Gain* 219

Your wind is the tender

To purchase insurance

That renders the splendor

Of greater endurance.

CHAPTER FOURTEEN

*Sexual Activity in the
Older Adult*   233

Attention to your cleanliness

Can increase your lover's friendliness.

And if you carefully self-inspect,

You'll improve your self-respect.

CHAPTER FIFTEEN

The Fountain of Age   *257*

I'll make myself stronger,

I'll make love still longer!

I'll summon the gumption

For my share of consumption.

WELCOME!

Someone may have given you this book or you might be standing in a bookstore perusing these pages and trying to decide whether to read on. So let me tell you more; and also, let me introduce myself. I'm Dr. Zinberg; and although I have published a number of medical papers, I've never written a book before. That notwithstanding, I felt compelled to write *Win In the Second Half* for my patients—and for you and your loved ones. This book will acquaint you with the many splendors that loom on your aging horizon; and even more importantly, it will help you deal with some of the problems that are hitched to the same wagon.

Every one of us will get old or die young. However, when accurately counted, we find that neither the term "old" nor "age" is a four-letter word. New discoveries have made for a much greater understanding of the so-called aging process. Our better appreciation of this process makes the information in this book of enormous importance, both to you as an individual and to our society in general.

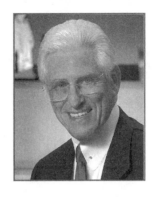

Almost all of us are aware that the effects of the baby boomer bang on the demographics of our country will be astounding. By the year 2010, there may be more people in this country between the ages of 54 to 74 than between the ages of 24 to 34; and by the year 2050, there may be more than one million people over the age of one hundred years. This, together with the remarkable achievements we've witnessed in medical science, particularly in the field of genetics, is likely to catalyze an incalculable increase in longevity for many if not most of us. During the next twenty years, the number of people in their seventies and eighties, and even in their nineties, is likely to increase exponentially. Many of you presently in your forties and fifties will have a much longer life than you might have anticipated and certainly longer than that of prior generations.

In short, more of us will age; and more of us will age even more. That's good and bad news. While this good news should give us many reasons to rejoice, the bad news should give us some important reasons to be concerned.

It's quite possible that as you age, you will encounter chronic disease, dwindling mental ability, and a decrease in physical strength, as well as a decrease in the acuity of each of your senses—taste, touch, smell, hearing, and eyesight. A great deal of how much of this happens to you and how soon it may happen to you is genetically determined; but virtually every authority agrees that genetics is not the only determinant of how you will age. In fact, it accounts for fifty percent or less of the process.

Fifty percent or more of how you age and how long you will live will be determined by environmental factors—the air you breathe, the food you eat, the amount of physical and mental exercise you get, and the like. Genes may load your gun, but your environment pulls the trigger. Much of this is under your control. You determine the food you eat and the exercise you do. Your choice of lifestyle makes up the greater part of your environment; and the right choices can delay or even reverse many of the effects of aging.

If you've made a series of bad choices, you must believe this: it's not too late—it really isn't. No matter your age, you can get mentally and physically stronger, become more energetic, become more vigorous, become more resistant to disease, and have a much happier and healthier life. The information in this book is dedicated to help you achieve this—but the choice is yours. Today is the first day of the rest of your life and you can decide what you want that life to be like. If you want to win in the second half or even in the last five years of your life, you can do it and the information contained herein will help you.

If you thumb through the pages, you will see that it has been written as a story involving people like you, your loved ones, your friends, and your neighbors. Conversational script is used to form a series of lectures and demonstrations at a community center. The expert presenting these discussions is the "not so fictional" Dr. Zinney, as portrayed by me. He humorously insinuates his knowledge of aging into the minds of his audience and teaches the participants how they can modify their own aging process. Serious and complex scientific information is simplified and further illuminated throughout the book as Zinney answers sometimes penetrating questions asked by members of his audience.

The practical questions asked helped him (me again) clarify some of the more scientifically complicated parts of the subject matter. The occasional illustrations, poems, rap ditties, and jokes produce still greater clarity.

The importance of this format and the reason for its selection is a direct result of what my patients have taught me in the privacy of the examination room during the last thirty-five years. I have learned that people are far more likely to make good decisions and stick with them when they thoroughly understand the scientific fundamentals underlying their concerns. Simply stated, when you understand something, you are more apt to believe it. If you believe it, you are more apt to embrace the tenets flowing out from it. To that end, *Win In the Second Half* carefully and plainly elucidates the scientific basis of the different aspects of aging. You will learn about the cellular and molecular nature of your mental and physical make-up and how the process of aging affects it. More importantly, you will learn how to beneficially alter these

changes through a detailed and thorough discussion of metabolism, diet, nutrition, herbs, supplements, and exercise.

Facts, both new and old, are affirmed and myths are deftly dispelled. As you read on, you will come to appreciate the magnificent benefits that await you by following the simple, safe, and thoroughly enjoyable programs I recommend for mental and physical exercise. You'll be astonished to find how all of this can quickly affect everything from skin to sex.

As an aside, it may serve your purpose to imagine yourself as part of the audience. If you do, please don't hesitate to interrupt me with any questions that come to mind.

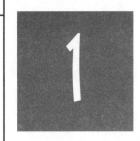

"Getting old isn't for sissies." *Bette Davis*

Health, like disease,

Can be contagious,

So infect yourself, please,

And read through these pages.

The problem

Sam awoke at 7:00 A.M. to a mournful groan. As he rubbed the sleep from his eyes, he heard a series of sobs coming from the bathroom. He stumbled out of bed and wearily trudged to the bathroom with an uncertain and unsteady gait. As usual, Sam had slept poorly. Three times during the night the urge to urinate sparked him from slumber. Each time he went to the toilet he experienced discomfort and difficulty in starting his urinary stream. Even worse was that the urine came out in a split fork that splashed on the rim of the toilet and on the floor requiring him to do a clean-up of the toilet and surrounding area or listen to the criticism of his wife, Sheila. "I love you darling, but don't spritz all over the bathroom. I know you're having prostate trouble; so if you can't pee straight, then for God's sake, sit down like I do."

This urinary problem had been bothering Sam for quite some time. He went to the doctor thinking that the frequent urination was a sign of diabetes but after thorough examination it was found that he had an enlarged prostate. He was placed on medication that seemed to be improving the condition but had to go through a series of tests to rule out cancer. The blood test, called a PSA, was slightly elevated so the doctor recommended a biopsy. The fear of cancer depressed him to no end. He was assured, however that the biopsy would not be painful and could be done in the office. What a surprise! The procedure consisted of putting a probe in his rectum that felt like a hot poker and then taking a series of punch biopsies of the prostate gland, each one producing a lancinating pain. Fortunately, the procedure was short; in retrospect it was not that bad, particularly since the biopsy was negative for cancer. But the doctor warned him that he would have to follow this condition with additional blood tests and possibly more biopsies in the future.

"Great," thought Sam. "What a wonderful thing to look forward to." Troubling him even more than pissing blood after the biopsy, was the recent change he noted in his sex life. Was it that he wasn't as interested at the age of sixty-five or was there something wrong with his penis? It didn't get as hard as it used to and sometimes died like an overripe banana before he could use it. "Praise be the Lord for Viagra," thought Sam.

Upon reaching the bathroom, Sam could see Sheila looking at herself in the mirror gasping, "Look at me! Look at the black rings under my eyes and the crow's feet in the corners. Look at me, Sam! I really, reeeelly need plastic surgery."

"You're a little loony to get so depressed over that. The way you were groaning I thought you were sick or in pain," Sam responded.

"Well, I am in pain. Just look at me! I really need something done."

"No, you don't. You look wonderful. Besides, cosmetic surgery costs a lot of money," said Sam.

"Well, Miriam is five years older than me. She had it done and she looks great."

"I really like Miriam. But you know—she's fifty-seven years old and looks seventy-seven. She had a double turkey neck before her surgery and now she just has one turkey neck. She should have paid half price. Miriam will never look or feel right until she loses some weight and stops smoking. Then she'll want plastic surgery again. She's at least thirty pounds overweight and has huge draping love handles that look like my mother's apron—not to mention her thighs look like the surface of the moon."

"You should talk! I'm really worried about you, Sam. Take a good look at your kangaroo pouch—you have trouble getting off the sofa! You're the typical couch potato. All you like to do is eat and watch TV. Ha! You're getting so round I'm afraid if you ever fell off the couch you'd roll 'till you starved to death."

"Very funny, Sheila. Ha, ha and ha again. But you know Miriam's husband Craig is no great shakes either. He's sixty-five and thinking of retiring. He says he thinks he has enough money and investments to live comfortably—if he doesn't live too long. The other day I noticed he seemed wobbly, as if he was losing his balance; and when we climbed a flight of stairs to the dentist he seemed really tired and short of breath. I asked him if he was all right and suggested he go to the doctor for a checkup. That went over like a lead balloon. He said he was just on a downer because of his older sister. She's seventy-six years old and suffers from arthritis and osteo-porosis. She's always dizzy and she's becoming very forgetful. Her physical discomfort causes her to do less and less; and so she gets weaker and weak-er. Now she has difficulty walking and climbing stairs. Add to that, her eye-sight and hearing are failing. And she's already had a hip replacement and four other surgeries. She's scared to death that she'll fall and break some-thing and end up in a nursing home. Her children, who almost never call her, have already suggested a nursing home. Boy, that really made her mad. She's a lonely and depressed woman. Her circle of friends is getting smaller because so many of them died," said Sam.

"I remember her," commented Sheila. "She was beautiful. A lot of women her age are full of wrinkles and the backs of their arms are as flabby as warm jello. Not her. I'm surprised she's deteriorating that rapidly."

"Getting old isn't for sissies—aches, pains, constipation, osteoporosis, and God knows what else," said Sam.

"A lot of it has to do with gravity," Sheila said.

"What do ya mean, gravity?" asked Sam.

"You know. Your boobs sag, your butt sags, the veins in your legs bulge—that sort of stuff. In one year Miriam's bladder, rectum, and uterus fell faster than Newton's apple and she had to have some kind of vaginal or pelvic suspender surgery," Sheila explained. "Things still don't work that good."

"Why is that?" questioned Sam.

Blushing from embarrassment, Sheila whispered, "Because she still has to put her finger in a private place to have a bowel movement."

"You're kidding me, aren't you?"

"No, I'm not. I wish I were. She'll probably need something more done. You can't go on like that."

"I don't know how she stands it," said Sam.

"Listen, Sam, we all have to get old or die young. Old isn't a four-letter word. It doesn't have to be bad. Take Jeff and Sue Kaplan. They're in their seventies and they play tennis three times a week. They belong to some

Fitness after Forty club. I'm sure there's a better way to take care of ourselves than the way we've been living. We need to improve our minds and our bodies. We have to make it happen," said Sheila.

"What do you know about it?" said Sam.

"Not much. But there's some doctor giving lectures each week at the community center. They're supposed to start tomorrow night. He wrote a book called *Win In the Second Half*. Maybe we should go."

"Personally, I think it's all a crock and a complete waste of time. He's probably just trying to sell his book," Sam replied.

"Well, I'm gonna go and I'm gonna drag your cute fat butt along with me. I'm also gonna tell Craig and Miriam about it. They might want to bring their niece, Bertha. She's forty-five and really went to pot since her divorce a few years ago. She needs help."

"I'm not gonna go," protested Sam. "I'd rather watch TV."

Sheila, in a most affirmative tone argued, "Yes, we are, we're going. I want to keep you around with me, Darling. I want us to have a healthier future together."

"Well, you may be going, but I'm not," he said.

The first night

The next night as Sam and Sheila entered the lecture hall at the community center, they predicted that the class would be poorly attended. They agreed that most folks don't want to know about the frailty of their future, and think they already have a pretty good idea about all the things they're doing wrong. They don't want to hear about how important it might be to make some changes in their lifestyle. After arguing with Sheila, Sam got his way and selected seats in the back row near the door. "If this lecture is as much bull as I think it's going to be, I want to be able to sneak out without making a fuss," he said. They saved three seats next to them for Miriam, Craig, and their niece Bertha. When their friends arrived, Sheila waved them over and they enthusiastically slid into the seats next to Sam.

Dr. Zinney

Martha Worthington, the director of education for the community center was at the podium and waited for the undercurrent of chatter to quiet down and the audience to be seated before going to the microphone, "For the next several weeks we will be treated to weekly lectures on aging and how we can do it better or, as Dr. Zinberg says it, how to 'Win In the Second Half.' Although our speaker is an experienced lecturer, he's told me that he always has sweaty palms before taking the microphone, and that he's embarrassed by exaggerated introductions—so, I'll be brief. Dr. Zinberg, or Dr. Zinney as he is often called, is a respected Internist who has had forty years of experience practicing Internal Medicine and in recent years has dedicated himself to the study of better aging. Without further adieu, I give you Dr. Zinney.

Despite an enthusiastic round of applause, Zinney was a little troubled by the unhappy expression on Sam's face. Much later, after Zinney and Sam became good friends, Sam confessed that his initial impression of Zinney was less than favorable. "I watched you jump on that podium," said Sam, "and I couldn't help thinking that you sure didn't look like Marcus Welby. I was right when I guessed you were in your late sixties, but you were much too flashy for my tastes. You dressed like a peacock; with all that silver hair and gold jewelry, you looked more like a Las Vegas gambler than a medical scholar— more likely to book a horse bet than give a medical lecture."

It's not too late

"Welcome, and thank you for coming here this evening," Zinney began. "What we will discuss tonight and over the ensuing weeks may be some of the most important information you will hear in regard to the rest of your life. At these meetings, we'll discuss the wish that all of us share. For our purpose, the letters of the word WISH will stand for 'Win In the Second Half.' We've all seen our favorite football or basketball team play the first half of a game poorly, and then stage a dramatic comeback to win the game in the second half. No matter how badly you've played the game of life in the first half, you too can stage a comeback and win in the second half. First you must WISH it, and then you must act on this wish to make it come true.

Muscle weakness or sarcopenia

"I know many of you think the damage is done; that it's too late to make a difference. Well, you're very lucky because you're very wrong. Whether frailty is the result of simple inactivity, poor eating habits, heart problems, lung problems, arthritis, or whatever; there is only one common denominator. That common denominator is muscle weakness.

"Between the ages of 45 and 60 we lose one percent of our muscle strength each year. This accelerates to an annual loss of one and a half percent of our muscle strength between the ages of sixty-five to seventy-five. Almost all of us here tonight are or will become significantly weaker at the age of seventy than we were at the age of forty. For some of you it will be dramatic. We can lose fifty percent or more of our muscle strength between the ages of forty-five and seventy-five.

Hard to believe? Well, it's true. The medical term for this age-related muscle deterioration is *sarcopenia*. The good news is that you might not be able to open that jar of jam or jelly and save yourself from some extra calories. The bad news is that, quite suddenly, you might not be able to get up from the toilet seat.

"On the other hand, the real good news is that recent studies in men and women between the ages of 80 and 90 who used resistance training two times a week showed exciting results. In just ten weeks they improved the strength in their legs by more than one hundred percent. Some of them even threw away their canes and walkers. Imagine!! These are people eighty and ninety years old. That's right!

Resistance training, like weight-lifting, made a huge difference. None of them became a Mr. Universe, but these results are indeed dramatic. In another recent study, a longer study, women placed on a strength-training program twice weekly for one year became biologically twenty years younger. They became seventy-five percent stronger, increased the bone density in their spine and hip areas, improved their balance, and became more active in their daily lives. They gained three pounds of muscle and lost three pounds of fat. Because a pound of muscle is much smaller in volume than a pound of fat, they were also slimmer and more shapely.

"So, you see, it's not too late—not by a long shot. You can keep the plaques in your arteries from getting bigger. You can make them smaller. You might even lose them entirely. You can make your arms and legs and your bones stronger. You can improve your energy level, your memory, your balance, your stamina, and your flexibility. You can feel better. You can look better. You will actually be better and you can accomplish all this with astonishing speed."

Self esteem

Craig waved his hand frantically until Dr. Zinney acknowledged him.

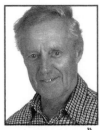

"That's all well and good, but what about our frame of mind?" asked Craig. "I would think that's as important or even more important than all this exercise stuff."

"You're right when you say it's important, but how you feel from a physical standpoint is often linked to how you feel about yourself," Zinney responded. "For many of us, successful aging has nothing to do with how many miles we can walk or whether we can do push-ups. It's related to a feeling of self worth or self-esteem. This feeling usually has its roots in our continued ability to make a contribution; whether it's to ourselves, to our business or employer, to our family or friends, to our community or our own garden, or through some form of volunteerism. This is often what makes us feel alive, appreciated, and productive. Nonetheless, it should be clear that the better our physical and mental abilities are; the better we will be able to make these contributions.

"These discussions will be informal. So ask questions or make comments at any time just as that last gentleman did. Just raise your hand and Martha or I will try to acknowledge you.

"Tonight we will discuss the biology of aging and how it applies to us. In subsequent discussions, we will try to understand how we can affect it and make it an enjoyable and fruitful process through changes in our lifestyle. We will see how we can avoid frailty, compress morbidity, and prolong our ability to live independently—to avoid the nursing home. We will go into detail about nutrition, diet, physical exercise, and mental exercise. We will explain the how, the why, the where, and the when. We'll even take field trips to exercise parlors and gyms for actual demonstrations. If you learn this information and you act upon it, you can Win In the Second Half. Now, let's talk a little about aging."

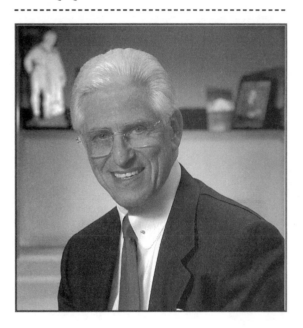

The human genome
May shape your dome,
But you're the crafter
Of what comes after.

The Beginning of Aging

Sheila noted a puzzled look on Sam's face and asked, "What's bothering you?"

"I don't get it," he replied. "What does Dr. Zinney mean when he talks about compressing morbidity?"

"He means that whether you live to be sixty or ninety that you stay healthy, independent, and functional during that time; and then, you drop dead. That's better than being frail and in a nursing home for your last fifteen years."

Increasing longevity

Zinney continued, "There are about three hundred theories on aging. While many have genuine scientific merit, they all need more study. But, what is clear is that we humans are living longer. About one hundred years ago, Otto Von Bismarck started the first retirement pension program. This program took effect at sixty-five years of age. At that time, the average lifespan was forty-five years of age; and since then, it has increased more than fifty percent. Scientists have good reason to believe that there may be an even greater increase in the next century. Sound crazy? Well, there's more. There's real truth in the old tongue-in-cheek adage that says, 'If I knew I was gonna live this long, I would have taken better care of myself.' It's conceivable that the average lifespan at the end of the next century will be 100 to 120 years with people maintaining the functionality we now observe in the average seventy-five year old."

Craig chuckled, "This guy Bismarck was smart. He probably selected the age of sixty-five because he knew almost no one would live long enough to collect."

Zinney continued, "The belief that you start to age from the minute you're born is interesting but inaccurate. Aging is a biologic balance of the increasing and decreasing rates of growth and repair. In humans, this rate changes between eleven years and twenty-five years of age. This is when the accelerating rate of growth and tissue repair begins to decelerate and aging begins. So you see, my friends, the saying, "life really begins at forty" is only half true. It only begins to *show* at forty.

Genetics and environment

"Your individual longevity depends in large part on your genetic make-up; but it is determined, to an even greater extent, by your environment. As an example, let's take two different kinds of flowers, one that thrives in sunlight and one that thrives in the shade. If we place them both in the sun, the one that does better in the shade may wither and die from excessive sunlight. Conversely, if you placed them both in the shade, the one that thrives in the sun may die. The nutritional content of our diet, the inhala-

tion of toxic fumes or tobacco smoke, our exposure to free radicals, a sedentary as opposed to an active physical existence—are all important factors. They can account for more than half of what you are or what you become. These factors all act on our genetic composition to determine the longevity and the morbidity, the suffering, that we will experience. The positive changes we can make in our environment will add life to our years as well as years to our lives. This is the WISH we must pursue; and, if we do, we can win in the second half."

"So now I'm supposed to believe I'm like a flower," Sam jested.

Sheila responded, "All he's saying is that what you do TO yourself or FOR yourself will make a difference, not only in how long you live but in the quality of your life. The last part is really important. For how ever long I live, whether it's for ten years or fifty years, I want to feel good and be healthy. It's all very logical."

Zinney continued, "Our longevity is a product of our genetic make-up and our environment. The genetic proclivity of some individuals to live longer is illustrated by those who have a family history of longer lifespans. On the other hand, there are those who have a family history of early death due to genetically-transmitted diseases, such as heart disease, neurological disorders, certain types of cancer, and diabetes. For example, it's believed that diabetes can accelerate the aging process by as much as thirty percent. Genetics can also be a determinant of our immune system. A good example of this is the Bubonic plague. Millions of people died while others, who were equally exposed, either failed to contract the disease or actually survived it.

Our cellular make-up

"Every one of us is made up of millions and millions of cells; and every cell in our body has a biologic time clock that determines how many times it can divide. The process of cell death and replacement continues at such a rapid rate that we are almost completely made anew each one to seven years—talk about makeovers. However, if every time a cell died it was replaced by a new cell, we would never change. We would look the same; we would be the same; we would never get older, and we would live forever. Fortunately or unfortunately, this is not the case. Each cell in our body has this time clock that limits the number of times it can divide and replace itself. When a cell can no longer divide to replace itself, it dies; and we lose cells. As more and more cells die and are not replaced, we age and then finally, we die."

DNA, chromosomes, and genes

As Dr. Zinney continued he projected a computer image on the screen [fig. 2A].

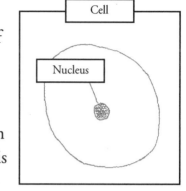

Fig 2A

"At the center of each cell in our body is the nucleus of the cell. Every cell in our body has this center, or nucleus, except our red blood cells.

"The nucleus of each one of our millions of cells contains our chromosomes [fig. 2B]. Our chromosomes

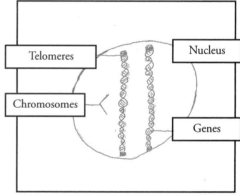

Fig 2B

contain the thousands and thousands of genes that determine our individual characteristics. The biologic time clock that I referred to is made up of tiny substances at the ends of each of our chromosomes. They're called *telomeres*. The longer the telomeres, the more times the cell can divide and therefore, the longer the life, potentially. With each cell division, the telomeres decrease in length. Shorter telomeres are associated with a decrease in the potential number of cell divisions and, consequently, a shorter cell life. A substance called telomerase regulates the length of these telomeres. The more telomerase, the longer the telomeres can maintain their length and the more often the cells can divide. On the flip side, it appears that cancer cells have an over-abundance of telomerase. If we develop the ability to inhibit specific kinds of telomerase we might develop a cure for some cancers at some time in the future.

"So you're saying that if this were all true, we could live forever," asked someone from the audience.

"In theory only," Zinney responded. "When George Bernard Shaw was asked in his later years if he had any advice for young people he said 'Don't try to live forever. You can't do it.' Decline in our physical reserve and some of our mental function is the inevitable result of aging, but we can positively and magnificently modify this process. And as I said earlier, the results of our efforts can be quickly achieved and truly dramatic. Successful aging requires our conscious effort to prevent illness, to stay physically and mentally fit, and to stay engaged with people and with life in general.

"The genome or genetic code of different animals and plants is an important determinant of longevity. For example, some turtles can live for an eternity, some varieties of rockfish live 150 years, and some trees live 5000 years. The longevity determinants in genetic codes are extremely complex. This is illustrated by the fact that ninety-eight percent of genes in humans and chimpanzees are the same; but humans live twice as long as chimps."

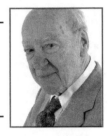

"Is this the DNA stuff that people talk about?" asked someone from the audience.

"Yes, this is our DNA," Zinney responded. "DNA is a very complex chemical that is different in each one of us. Although ninety-nine percent or more of genetic code may be identical from person to person, the one percent or less difference is more than enough to differentiate each one of us. To summarize all this, our DNA is in the nucleus of each cell. Within our DNA lie our chromosomes, our entire genetic code. The letters, DNA, stand for deoxyribonucleic acid; but it's of little importance that you remember the chemical name. The DNA in the nucleus of our cells manufactures the RNA that is outside the nucleus of the cell. RNA stands for ribonucleic acid. The RNA makes up the cytoplasm. That's the part of the cell outside the nucleus, the rest of the cell. The part of the cell outside of the nucleus is called the cytoplasm. Here's a simple diagram of a cell that helps explain what I mean," said Zinney as he projected a labeled picture on the screen [fig. 2C].

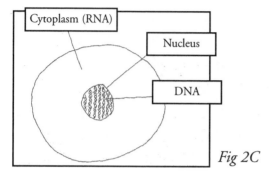

Fig 2C

"Here you can see a diagram of a cell. The nucleus contains DNA; and the RNA is outside the nucleus in the cytoplasm of the cell.

"In recent years, scientists have found ways to rearrange DNA. This involves very complicated techniques that splice chromosomes and infuse them into bacteria with the use of viruses. These techniques produce what is called *recombinant DNA*.

"Recombinant DNA can be used to alter the genetic code of a plant, animal, or human. Our knowledge of this process has already been used to produce special pharmaceuticals such as human insulin, to diagnose certain genetic diseases, to replace defective or disease causing genes, or to add protective genes. Some diseases are already treated this way and many more will be treated this way in the future.

"Now that scientists have completed the map of the human genome, there may be a dramatic acceleration of wonderful discoveries that will have a positive effect on longevity and morbidity. Altering the genetic code of certain worms, known as nematodes, has doubled their lifespan. Also, by altering the genetic code of the fruit fly, its lifespan was doubled; its resistance to heat and cold was improved; and its ability to mate increased tenfold."

Sam laughed and said, "What is it with this guy? He's talking about worms and a bionic fruit fly that became a sex maniac."

"Well, for sure Sam, you're no John F. Fruit Fly. I should only be that lucky," said Sheila. "But it could be fun to get our hands on some of those genes." Sam smiled in agreement.

Messengers

"It has recently been discovered that special proteins act as messengers that may activate or govern the activity of genes. Learning what these specialized proteins do may enable scientists to develop drugs that control genetic activities. Some agents that actually decrease blood vessel growth have already been discovered. In the future, we may treat cancer by depriving the cancer cells of blood. Other proteins increase blood vessel growth. They may have a beneficial effect in treating heart disease and other circulatory problems."

Stem cells

"Dr. Zinney, earlier, when you were talking about telomerase, you made mention of stem cells. There's been a lot of commotion about stem cells lately. Can you tell us what they are?" asked Miriam.

"Well, okay. I'm really glad you asked that question because the developments in stem cell research have the potential to improve the quality and length of life. They might dramatically change the way medicine is practiced. First, let's talk about the similarities stem cells have with our other cells. A stem cell, like any other cell in our body, has a nucleus. It contains all of our DNA. Our other cells have already differentiated into specialized cells like skin cells, muscle cells, bone cells, and the like. Stem cells are cells that have not yet specialized into these different types. All of us have stem cells but the more abundant sources are found in the early stages of the developing embryo and placenta. These less mature stem cells seem to have greater potential to specialize into a wider variety of different types of cells than more mature or adult stem cells.

"Scientists now have the ability to culture these stem cells outside of the body; and more recently, scientists developed functioning kidneys in mice with the use of stem cells. Just imagine if scientists could produce skin stem cells to treat burn victims or nerve stem cells to treat patients with spinal cord injuries or Alzheimer's disease. A whole host of other diseases might be treated this way. We're a long way from all this because a lot of research has to be done; but the potential is very exciting."

Stress

Zinney continued, "As we said earlier, your genetic make-up is not the only determinant of your physical and mental future. Environment is exceedingly important. The possum is a good animal example. Its lifespan is precariously short. When experimentally taken to an island where there was less predatory stress, the lifespan of these animals almost doubled when compared to those subjected to the predatory stress of their previous habitat. This experiment suggests that stress may have an important effect, not only on the quality of life, but also on the length of life.

Diet

"It's also been shown that caloric restriction can increase longevity. In one experiment, the lifespan of mice was increased by thirty percent by simply restricting calories. These mice even performed better than their counterparts. They moved faster, fatigued less, and were more capable of negotiating a maze. This goes along with the finding in nature that birds that fly faster usually fly longer and live longer."

Craig raised his hand and asked, "Dr. Zinney, how much caloric restriction are you talking about in terms of us humans by comparison to the mice you're talking about?"

"It would equate to about 1700 calorie per day for an average-sized person, but understand that this is just an approximation. While caloric restriction might prove to be beneficial to human performance and longevity, the precise amount of caloric restriction is not at all clear," Zinney responded.

"I would starve on 1700 calories," said Craig.

Free radicals and antioxidants

"You wouldn't starve; but your diet would likely be that of a vegetarian. There's a lot of merit to eating more vegetables. As you probably know, many of them are an excellent source of antioxidants, which we believe play an important role in retarding the aging process. Let me explain. Free oxygen radicals are thought by many to be the major culprit that causes cell damage and aging. They are a result of the normal metabolism of oxygen in our bodies. They are also found as pollutants in our air and can be increased by excessive sun exposure.

"Some believe that cigarette smoking and diets high in animal fat can further increase the accumulation of free radicals. An appealing analogy is that free radicals cause oxidative cell damage much like the free radicals in the atmosphere cause iron to rust. In other words, they are believed to cause the cells of our bodies to rust, then to age, and to die.

"The accumulation of these free radicals has been associated with a wide range of disorders, from cancer and cardiovascular diseases to skin wrinkles. Antioxidants, such as vitamin A, beta-carotene, vitamin E, vitamin C, selenium, and others, scavenge these free radicals and prevent their accumulation. These antioxidants are abundantly present in dark green vegetables, carrots, fish, milk, eggs, and asparagus. The need or value of antioxidant supplements is controversial, but we'll talk more about diet and nutrition later."

A casually dressed man, who appeared to be in his mid-fifties, asked, "What about our brain power—you know, our memory? Don't antioxidants help that too?"

"Good question. They might! And there's more you can do, but we're out of time for tonight. That's what we'll talk about next week. We'll call it our Memory and Mental Muscles," said Zinney. "Thank you for coming tonight and if you think of any questions between now and next week, bring them along and I'll try to answer them."

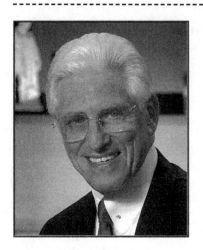

3

Plaques and tangles,
Tangles and plaques,
Our mind it mangles,
And some it cracks.

Our Mental Muscle

The lecture hall was filled a few minutes before the designated starting time and more people were still filing in. Ms. Worthington signaled her assistant to get some extra chairs as Zinney took the microphone.

"Welcome to all of you. I'm glad to see some familiar faces from last week and pleased to see so many new faces. For those of you who don't know me, I'm Dr. Zinberg; but as I've told my friends from last week, you can call me just plain Zinney. Tonight we're going to talk about our mental and memory muscles—both the good news and the bad news. There's no doubt that physical changes will occur in our brain with advancing age but before getting into that, we should all get a general understanding of the brain and how it works. Scientists themselves have only a very small understanding of how the brain works. There are many more mysteries yet to be solved.

The brain and the nervous system

"During the early stages of embryonic development, our cells receive a signal that determines their differentiation and specialization. Some cells become heart cells; some become lung cells; some become bone cells, and so on. The specialized cells that make up our brain and the rest of our nervous system are called neurons. If you look at the diagram I've projected on the screen, you can see that these neurons have long branches called dendrites [fig. 3A].

"These dendrites (or branches) connect with other neurons. The connection between one neuron and another is

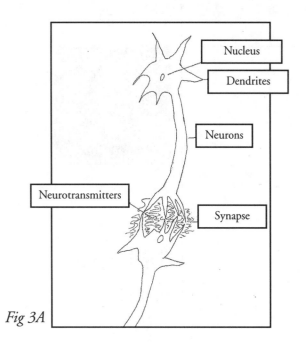

Fig 3A

called a synapse. Messages are transmitted from one neuron to another neuron across these connections, or synapses. Chemicals produced in the brain and at these synapses help to transmit the messages. They're called neurotransmitters. That's how messages pass from one neuron to another. That's how we think, how we move, and how we recall or remember things."

Neurons and synapses

"Dr. Zinney, John Kinder here. I'm sorry, but I still don't think I got all that."

"Well let me take a crack at clarifying it," Zinney replied. "The brain and the nervous system are made up of specialized cells called neurons, or nerve cells; these cells have branches called dendrites. Each cell communicates with other nerve cells by transmitting messages along their branches to other connected nerve cells. The synapse is where the nerve cells connect. It's like an electrical circuit. What we now realize is that both mental and physical exercise can improve circulation to the brain and the branching and connecting of these cells. This improves mental ability.

Glial cells

"There are billions of these neuron cells as well as billions of other kinds of cells in the nervous system, such as glial cells. Glial cells have long been regarded as little more than structural supporting cells in the brain; however, recent research suggests they may play an important role in increasing the growth of dendrites and the number of synapses. This information may have a significant impact on our understanding of brain diseases and the treatment of these disorders as we forge into the future.

Our aging minds

"Studies have shown that about one-half of our mental ability is genetically determined and that this genetic influence persists into old age. This is true for memory, problem solving, reading, writing skills, and the speed at which we think. But the other half is actually determined by our lifestyle—our diet, our exercise habits, and our mental initiative. But we'll talk more about this later.

"With progressive aging, there may be a decrease in the number of neurons, dendrites, and synapses (or connections). This can result in a decrease in spatial orientation, in deductive reasoning, and in short-term memory—that's the bad news. The good news is—that there are some things the brain does better as it ages; and also, that the bad news can be delayed, compensated for, and even, in part, reversed."

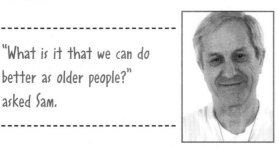

"What is it that we can do better as older people?" asked Sam.

Judgment

"We can make judgments involving life's experience better as we age. Some people call this wisdom—using the knowledge we've gained from experience to solve problems. Every success and every failure we've had is an experience. Some of us have learned a great deal from these experiences and can recall and apply them. In other instances, we can't actually recall the experience because it's buried deep within that magnificent computer called our brain. Here it produces a gut feeling or automatic reflex that often serves us every bit as well as if we could recall it. Younger people often discount these gut feelings because they're taught to justify their decisions with logical analysis. But they don't have as much life experience as we do. We are sometimes frustrated by what appears to be analysis-paralysis and the reluctance of younger people to accept our judgment. But we must appreciate that it is precisely that type of analysis that programmed our own mental computer during our own youthful days.

"It's true that some of the experience we've accumulated over the years may no longer be of value today because of the advent of new technology. But life experiences with interpersonal relationships haven't changed. Studies designed to test the ability of people to solve difficult interpersonal life problems showed that older people scored higher than younger people. It appears that although we may remember less, we may understand more. We may have a better understanding of broad concepts even though we experience more difficulty remembering specific details.

Forgetfulness

"Many of us note that with advancing age we don't think as fast as we used to. We don't process new information as well. We forget what jokes or stories we've told to people, and we repeat ourselves over and over again. We forget where we left our glasses or the keys to our car; we forget a word or a name and become convinced that dementia is looming on our doorstep. Well, you'll hear me say this over and over again as we go forward, *Remember this—you've been forgetting things all your life.*

Dementia and Alzheimer's

"Each of us knows someone with multi-infarct dementia or with Alzheimer's disease. We imagine that one of these dreaded disorders will pull us into that horrible dimension. These fears are often exaggerated. About ten percent of people over the age of sixty-five may become afflicted, while ninety percent do not. In more advanced age groups, people between the ages of eighty-five and one hundred, the incidence can increase to as much as fifty percent. But even here, it is important to know that some people experience significantly less impairment than others.

"Because some of us may have family members with this disorder, we become convinced it is our destiny to also be afflicted. While it's true that genetics play a role in early-onset Alzheimer's disease, it's also clear that genetics play a much smaller role in later years. Dietary and nutritional factors, infections, and exposure to toxic fumes have been incriminated. Numerous other things in our environment that have yet to be identified or discovered may prove to play a significant role in determining the presence or absence, as well as the severity, of this disease. Here again your lifestyle can be the important determining factor."

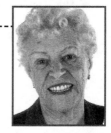

"Dr. Zinney, my name is Thelma Magnus. I'd like to know what actually happens to the brain in Alzheimer's disease."

"Well, Thelma, we're not exactly sure. But I'll tell you what we think we know about it. Autopsy studies on the brains of people who have had Alzheimer's disease reveal an abnormal accumulation of protein plaques. They're called amyloid plaques. As the disease progresses, tangles also develop in the brain cells. It is believed that the accumulation of these plaques and tangles is responsible for the disease; but the precise role that they play is not completely understood. Strangely, these plaques have also been found in the autopsies of some people who have had no symptoms or signs of Alzheimer's disease while they were alive. Some studies have suggested that the ingestion of aluminum might be a factor—like the aluminum in some of the antacids that you might take for indigestion or the aluminum in cookware; but the jury is still out on aluminum. Exactly how or why these plaques develop and accumulate still puzzles the scientific community," Zinney replied.

"Am I to understand that we can't be sure about Alzheimer's without an autopsy?" asked Thelma.

"While the finding of these plaques at autopsy is considered the gold standard for diagnosis, most authorities believe the diagnosis can be accurately established in more than ninety percent of cases by psychological and neurological testing. These tests seek to identify cognitive impairments and structural changes that appear to be good predictors of early Alzheimer's," Zinney replied. "Recently the use of a chemical marker combined with a PET scan (positron emission tomography) has been used to identify early changes that seem to be highly accurate in diagnosing and predicting the likelihood of developing Alzheimer's disease. An enormous amount of research is being conducted on this disease and breakthroughs often seem just moments away. Recently, a protein has been found in the blood of patients with this disease that shows great promise as a diagnostic marker. Also, a vaccine that showed excellent results in animals will soon be tested on humans. Genetic studies appear to have identified five genes on chromosome number ten that are relevant to Alzheimer's disease. Of more immediate interest, anti-inflammatory drugs and a number of other pharmacological agents appear to delay the progress of Alzheimer's disease. So you see, there is real hope for those who become afflicted. We predict that this disease, like so many others before it, will be conquered.

"A friend of mine has spent the better part of his professional life doing research on Alzheimer's disease and has participated in the discovery of those abnormal genes on chromosome ten. He was particularly motivated because two of his family members suffered from this horrid disease.

"But the real tragedy was further underscored when he discovered that he himself had some of the early signs of this disease. Nonetheless, he has bravely and furiously continued with his research. He wrote a poem about Alzheimer's and dedicated it to his patients and their families.

"He called it 'Plaques and Tangles.'
It goes like this:

Plaques and tangles
       Tangles and plaques
Our mind it mangles
       And some it cracks.

On chromosome ten
       We've found real hope.
We'll search yet again
       While all of us cope.

A vaccine or drug
       We'll soon discover
From the genes we debug
       Or might uncover.

We'll decipher a cure
       From the code of creation,
So, strive to endure
       While we seek God's salvation."

"You mentioned anti-inflammatory drugs. I guess you mean
the kind used to treat
arthritis. Why would they
help Alzheimer's disease?" asked Sam.

"I'm glad you asked," replied Zinney. "Some students of the disease believe there is a significant inflammatory component that occurs in the brain of patients with Alzheimer's. Some theorize that anti-inflammatory drugs, like those used to treat arthritis, can delay the progress or onset of the disease. Also, there are a number of medications intended to improve memory and many more on the researcher's drawing boards.

"On another note, there are also some interesting surgical approaches to this disease currently under investigation. One makes use of the apron of fatty material in the abdomen, known as the omentum, as a covering for the brain. This has been associated with astonishing improvement in some patients. Exactly how or why this works is not clear; but research is in progress. So you see, hope springs eternal from many sources."

"One more question, Dr. Zinney. What is that other kind of dementia you mentioned?" asked Thelma.

"You must mean my earlier reference to multi-infarct dementia. That's a form of dementia that might be caused by the death of brain cells resulting from the deprivation of blood flow to the brain. It's not the same as Alzheimer's disease."

"You mean it's like a stroke?"

"Yes, Thelma. It's caused by strokes, sometimes multiple tiny strokes that may even go unnoticed by the victim," Zinney answered.

Depression, loss of esteem, distraction

"Since we know that dementia can be gradual in onset, the first sign of weakness we perceive in ourselves causes many of us to become depressed. We begin to lose confidence in our capacities. This loss of self-esteem acts as a catalyst that can cause a further depreciation of self-efficacy or self-confidence.

"While most of us under the age of eighty-five don't suffer from dementia, we indiscriminately interpret the forgetfulness that normally comes with aging as the beginning of this dementia. If you forget where you put your keys, it's not terribly important; we all do that. If you forget what the keys are for and to whom they belong, it could be important. If you forget where you put your hat and your glasses, it's not terribly important. But if you put them in the freezer, it could be important. All of us forget the names of some of the people we meet; that's not serious. But if we forget the names of our children or grandchildren, that could be serious. A story I like to tell in this regard goes :

"A ninety-five year old lady and her ninety year old kid sister had lunch every single day on the same park bench for twenty years. One day the younger lady said to her older sister, 'Darling, there's something that has been bothering me for the last two weeks and I've been ashamed to mention it.'

'You shouldn't be ashamed to tell your older sister anything. Tell me what's bothering you. Maybe I can help,' replied the older lady.

'Well, for the last two weeks I've been trying and trying but I can't remember your name,' said the younger woman. 'Please remind me.'

'Sure,' said the older sister. She took a pencil and a piece of paper from her purse and when poised to write, she asked, 'How soon do you need it?'

"Unlike the sisters in this joke, too often we needlessly harbor and nurture inappropriate fears; and in some instances, we become thoroughly possessed by them even though the odds are so much in our favor. The famous words of FDR, 'There is nothing to fear but fear itself' can be judiciously applied here. Sometimes our mental lapses are due to simple impatience, causing a lack of focus or concentration. In other cases, it may be because we are more easily distracted and need more privacy to assimilate certain types of information. In still other cases, we may have taken stored information so much for granted that we forget it. While mental ability and creativity may go unimpaired in some of us despite our advancing age, you can't let a little forgetfulness get you down. Let me repeat this: we've been forgetting things since we were born."

Creativity

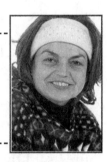

"I've always been led to believe that invention and creativity wane dramatically with age," Sheila said.

"That's a very popular misconception," Zinney replied. "History is replete with examples that disprove that myth. Let me amplify that a little," Zinney continued. "Many innovations in mathematics have been developed by people in their third and fourth decades of life, and many innovations in physics and engineering have been developed by people in their fourth and fifth decades of life. Still, many discoveries were made in the field of biology; and numerous works in history, art, and literature were produced by people later in life. Let me give you some actual examples:

- Michelangelo designed and worked on the dome of Saint Peter's Basilica from age seventy-two until his death at age eighty-eight.

- Freud published some of his most important theories between the ages of sixty-five and seventy.

- Georgia O'Keefe painted some her best works in her late sixties and early seventies.

- Grandma Moses (Anna Mary Robertson) was a farmer's wife for most of her life. She began her painting career in her late seventies.

- Frank Lloyd Wright was ninety-one years old when he designed the Guggenheim Museum.

- Stradivari made his best violins in his early nineties.

- Galileo wrote his most important scientific theories at the age of seventy-four.

- Marie Curie won a Nobel prize in her mid-forties for isolating radium. She surely would have continued to make contributions in later life were it not for her untimely death from leukemia.

- Sarah Bernhardt continued her creative acting on the stage into her late seventies despite a leg amputation in her sixties.

- Picasso painted masterpieces at the age of eighty.

- Alfred Hitchcock directed *The Birds* and *Frenzy* in his 60s and 70s.

- Dr. Seuss was in his 80s when he wrote *You're Only Old Once.*"

"But these people were always creative geniuses," Sheila argued.

"In my opinion there is a genius buried within each and every one of us, it just has to be awakened. Inspiration is the father of creativity and we must open our minds to recognize and accept inspiration. The examples I've given just scratch the surface of the history of creativity and what it can teach us. It is more important for us to understand that we use creativity in solving every problem and in making every decision throughout the day. We develop ways to accomplish things in our everyday lives that make it easier for each of us to do certain tasks. This is the thought process of creativity. This creativity can take the form of a better way for a teacher to present a subject to the class, or even what necktie to wear with a certain suit, or what necklace to wear with a certain dress.

"Complacency is the enemy of creativity. People lose their creativity when they stop caring about things, when they are less concerned about the outcomes of events, when they convince themselves that they can't influence the course of events, when they adopt the complacent attitude of 'what will be, will be.' But each and every one of us can make a difference. Whatever we do, or don't do, can affect the outcome of certain events. Clearly, in many cases, the magnitude of the effect we have on any given event might be miniscule but one cannot always accurately make that judgment before trying. We must avoid the laziness of complacency. We must energize ourselves to think and be creative.

Brain growth factor

"As we age, brain function can be maintained and even improved. There's a chemical substance called *brain growth factor* produced in the brain that can be increased with physical and mental exercise. Physical exercise appears to increase neuronal dendrite formation and cerebral circulation.

"Mental challenges such as memory games, crossword puzzles, reading, and problem solving of almost any kind are all examples of mental exercise that seem to increase the branching and connections of brain cells.

Varying mental activities and introducing novel or new tasks are particularly helpful. Endeavors such as volunteering on an advisory committee, taking part in discussion groups, taking classes in art or literature, or anything of particular interest to a given individual can enhance the production of brain growth factor.

New skills

"Developing new skills, such as becoming computer literate, surfing the web and using e-mail, can be mentally stimulating as well as enjoyable. The idea that you can't teach an old dog new tricks is erroneous. One of the most important things you can do as you age is to learn new skills. Someone who is a champion bridge player or a chess master can maintain this skill well into their later years. While maintaining these skills is excellent mental exercise, it is even better exercise to learn a new skill.

"Scientists used to believe that after full development of the brain it gradually and irreversibly atrophies over a period of years and that this deterioration could not be halted or reversed. We now know that this concept is incorrect. Both physical and mental exercise can increase brain growth factor, brain size, and mental ability."

"Wasn't there some study done on taxi drivers that proved that?" Miriam asked.

"Yes indeed, among many others," Zinney responded. "In a large metropolitan area scientists measured the brain size of newly hired taxi drivers. Two years later, after the drivers learned the traffic routes associated with their new job, they measured their brain again and found a significant increase in size. The mental challenge of learning this new material actually increased their brain size.

Distraction and concentration

"Many young people can study calculus while listening to hard rock. Us older folks are more easily distracted and need more solitude to maintain our focus. This is particularly true in learning complex material. When attempting to learn new material or develop a new skill, take care to avoid distraction. It is the ability to concentrate that appears to wane with age just as muscle power may weaken with age and disuse.

"And just as you can strengthen your muscles by physical exercise, you can strengthen your power of concentration with practice. We must work at it. Most people who exercise regularly don't really like to exercise. They just think they like to exercise because they love the way it makes them feel. Most people who concentrate and study hard don't like it while they're doing it, but they love the sense of accomplishment, the feeling of self-satisfaction, and the way the power of knowledge makes them feel. As we age, we get lazy in terms of physical exercise and lazy in terms of concentration. Just as we must motivate ourselves to do physical exercise, we must will ourselves to concentrate; we must make ourselves concentrate.

"The following story is an example: Two brothers, ages 90 and 95, were riding in car. The younger brother was driving.

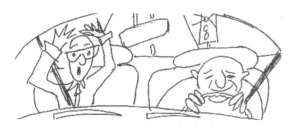

"'You just passed through a red light. You'd better be careful,' said the older brother. The younger brother continued driving without acknowledging his older brother's concern.

A short while later the older brother exclaimed, 'You passed through another red light. We're gonna get a ticket if you're not careful.' The younger brother continued driving, again without a reply, and then passed through yet a third red light.

The older brother screamed, 'Are you crazy? You wanna get us killed? You went through three red lights in a row!'

To which the younger brother replied, 'I'm sorry. I thought you were driving.' "

Improvement

"Serious scientific experiments have now demonstrated that changes in environment, the introduction of novelty, mental exercise, and physical exercise can actually increase dendritic sprouting, increase synapses, increase blood flow to the brain cells, and improve cognition or mental ability. The use of estrogens in women and the use of antioxidants have also been shown to be of value in preserving brain function. On the other hand, stress, the avoidance of variety, and couch potato kind of inactivity are likely to be associated with a more rapid decline in mental ability.

"Actually, your memory can begin to decline after you reach the age of sixteen years. Moreover, it can decline at a rate of one percent a year between the ages of forty and seventy years. This can translate into a loss of thirty percent of your memory related skills. However, my good friends, we can do something about it. We can do a lot to preserve and even improve our brain function with lifestyle changes. A healthful diet, physical exercise, and the proper mental exercise can improve your mental ability and even your memory by twenty years. That means that a person who is seventy-five years old can improve his or her mental ability to what it was when he or she was fifty-five years old.

"Stay engaged with life, with current events, with all that's going on around you. Don't let anybody tell you that you can't do it. You can learn to play bridge, paint a picture, sculpt a statue, or write a book or an essay. Don't let anybody rob you of your self-esteem by convincing you that you can't do something. You can do it. But you, and only you, can do it. First, you must be a champion to yourself. Pick your dreams, hang on to them, and pursue them with vigor. Albert Einstein was right when he said 'Imagination is more important than knowledge.' But knowledge is also important and it can be a powerful

ally. So we must constantly try to improve and increase our fund of knowledge."

Sam, now becoming more interested in the discussion, asked,

"Dr Zinney, you talked about the need to make ourselves concentrate. You mentioned the need for novelty, variety, patience, and the need for avoiding distraction when trying to learn something complex or new. But that still doesn't tell me how to improve my memory."

The constituents of memory

"Well, you're right. The things you mentioned: the need to avoid distraction, the need for variety, and the need to be patient with yourself are all very important in improving your learning skills and your retention of information. But before getting into actual mental exercises, we might be well served to learn something about the constituents of memory.

"In order to remember something, you must *learn* that something first. Next, you must *store* the information and then you must be able to *recall* it.

Learning, storing, and recalling are the three main constituents or phases of memory. They work hand-in-hand.

Rules of remembering

"The better you learn and understand something, the better you store that information. The more often you repeat something you've learned, the better you reinforce the storage. Then, the more often you recall it, the easier it becomes to recall that information and the more it strengthens the storage of that information.

"As an example, many of you can remember the phone number of a friend or a loved one. The more frequently you dial the number, the easier it is to remember. The less frequently you dial it, the harder it becomes to recall. Remembering things is made easier by following four important rules. The four important rules are: *repetition*, *perseverance*, *patience*, and *belief* in yourself. No matter how often you fail, you must repeat, persevere, have patience with yourself, and believe in yourself, because YOU CAN DO IT.

"Well, folks, we are out of time tonight. I'll look forward to seeing you next week when we'll try some of the actual exercises we can use to improve our mental abilities."

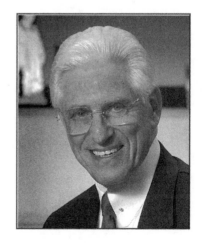

4

Your mind is your mate;

You govern its state.

You open its gate,

When you concentrate.

Brainaerobics and Mindercises

Ms. Worthington had a bad case of the flu and asked Dr. Zinney to act as the master of ceremonies for tonight's meeting. Being a giant ham, Zinney had little problem in accepting his role.

"Tonight we're going to discuss techniques for learning and remembering. Many of us age with no perceptible deficit in our memory, learning skills, or creativity. However, for those of us who feel these talents are fading, there are exercises that will improve and even rehabilitate our mental abilities. For lack of a better term, we'll call these exercises, *brainaerobics* and *mindercises*. As we enter this phase of our discussions, it will be important for all of us to remember the four rules for learning: *repetition*, *perseverance*, *patience* with ourselves, and *belief* in ourselves.

"We also learned last week that there are three aspects to remembering: *learning*, *storage*, and *recall*. These three must be integrated if we're going to be effective. We must learn something before we can store that something and then we must be able to recall that something in order to use the information. As we go forward, it also seems worth repeating that regardless of age, nobody's memory is perfect. Those of you who had a photographic memory when you were younger may be finding yourselves a little short on film these days. But remember, we've been forgetting things all our lives.

"Our memory for things that happened years ago is often better than our ability to remember whom we had lunch with yesterday. This decrease in short-term memory may be, in part, due to a lack of concentration. Also, as previously discussed, and for reasons that are not entirely clear, we are more easily distracted as we age and need more solitude or privacy to concentrate effectively.

"Again, we've been forgetting things all our lives, so don't get discouraged. Be patient with yourself and persevere. Don't sabotage your learning process. Allow yourself the luxury of a quiet place that is free from distraction. This is particularly important when trying to learn something new or complex. We will separate this discussion into three phases as follows: learning new material, simple memory exercises, and practical ways to remember things that effect everyday real-life situations.

Use your senses

"Many of us learn things by hearing a lecture or listening to a recording. Others learn more by reading—by looking at the written words and visual aids, such as pictures or diagrams. Activities such as rewriting the material to be learned or saying the material out loud can reinforce our ability to store information and to recall it. If you role-play or say the material aloud, you can concentrate on the information and hear it at the same time. Reading information, writing it, and saying it aloud over and over again further entrenches the information in your storage bin and improves your ability to recall it. The more you recall and rehearse information, the more likely you are to retain the information in your long-term memory.

Learning new material

"Some material can be difficult to assimilate because of its complexity. In such instances, it can be helpful to write an outline. Then, learn the headings of the outline by writing them, reading them, and saying them aloud. After learning the headings, learn the material in each section using the same technique. Demonstrate to yourself that you know a section or two before proceeding. When you've completed all of the sections, take it from the top, as they say in show biz, and review the entire outline. Write it, read it, say it, and hear it. Repetition-repetition-repetition.

"This technique can be used to understand particularly complicated things like insurance policies, contracts, or directions on how to operate devices, like a cell phone or VCR. During the process of learning the material, write key questions about the material.

When you're confident that you've learned the material, you can test yourself with these questions.

"Exercises like this can improve your learning ability and your memory. Some of you may think they're mindless, but believe me, they really work. Practicing these learning exercises and the memory exercises we will discuss later tonight can improve brain function. They may increase the branching and the connecting of brain cells, improve circulation to the brain, and increase the production of brain growth factor. All this may result in an astonishing improvement in mental ability. As I said, sometimes memory can be improved to that of a person twenty years younger than you are."

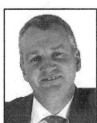

Someone from the audience asked, "But what if someone twenty years younger than I also practiced with these exercises? Could I still equal him or her in memory ability?"

"Not likely," Zinney responded. "But that doesn't diminish the value of doing these exercises. The benefit that YOU achieve is the thing that's important here, and those benefits can be absolutely amazing. So, let's get on with learning the exercises!

Memory exercises

"The first exercise makes use of an ordinary deck of playing cards. Place two cards face down as shown on the projection screen [fig. 4A].

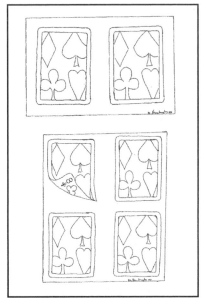

Fig 4A

"Look at what cards they are, place them face down again, and see if you can remember them. Repeat this with four cards, placing two on top and two below. Try to name the four cards, then turn them face up and see if you're correct.

"When you have mastered the ability to remember four cards, try two rows of three cards each. When you have conquered remembering two rows of three cards each, try three rows of three cards each, and so on.

Association

"Sometimes using an association technique will help you remember sequences. For example, let's say that the three cards on the top row are the king of clubs, the ten of hearts, and the queen of diamonds. A simple story that would help one to recall their order might go as follows: The king of the club gave ten valentines to his queen who was dressed in diamonds. Developing this kind of association is often fun and improves your ability to be innovative. Some sequences lend themselves to developing an association more easily than others. On other occasions, attempting to develop an association is more difficult and we are better served by trying to learn the sequence with raw perseverance and repetition. Nonetheless, attempting to develop this kind of association is fun and might even improve your ability to innovate.

Memorizing poems or jingles

"Another good exercise is memorizing short poems or jingles. This can be done by memorizing one line at a time using the learning technique of reading, writing, then reciting. I would suggest that the poems be no longer than six to eight lines to start. If you're successful, then you can try longer poems. Books of poems are available in libraries and in almost any bookstore. This is not only a good exercise and a lot of fun, it's also very educational. Imagine the look on the face of a friend when you recite poetry, particularly if it's appropriate for a specific event like a birthday or a graduation. Poems with a memorable tempo and rhyme scheme are especially appropriate because the tempo and the rhyming will assist you in remembering them.

"Short musical jingles that rhyme are not very popular anymore; but they are excellent as memory exercises because they have tempo, rhyme, and usually a catchy tune that can aid the recall. Some good oldies that fit the bill are the old Pepsi Cola, Rinso, and Oscar Mayer Wiener jingles. Also, some catchy little tunes like 'Mares Eat Oats' can work the same way.

"They're good exercises that can be a lot of fun and have the additional benefit of strengthening the voice and improving a person's ability to articulate. Scores of them are readily available on the Internet.

"Come on. All of you sing along." Zinney then proceeded to sing,

> *"Rinso white,*
> *Rinso bright,*
> *Happy little wash day song."*

"Come on, you folks. Get into it and sing along. All together now." While almost no audience participation was evident at first, Zinney cheerfully urged them on. "You probably never heard that one. Let's try another one." The audience responded by building to a crescendo as more and more participated until almost everyone was singing.

"Pepsi Cola hits the spot,
Twelve full ounces, that's a lot.
Twice as much for a nickel, too.
Pepsi Cola is the drink for you."

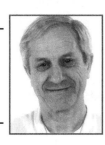

"That's a very old oldie," said Sam. "You couldn't buy the empty can for a nickel today."

"Now, let's try the Oscar Meyer jingle," urged Zinney.

"I wish I were an Oscar
Meyer wiener,
That is what I really want to be.
'Cause if I were an Oscar
Meyer wiener,
Everyone would be in love
with me.

"That was great, folks. Now, let's try 'Mares Eat Oats.'

"Mares eat oats and does eat oats
And little lambs eat ivy.
A kid'll eat ivy, too,
Wouldn't you?
If the words sound queer
And funny to your ear
A little bit jumbled and jivey—
Sing mares eat oats and does
*   eat oats*
And little lambs eat ivy.

Mares eat oats and does eat oats
And little lambs eat ivy.
A kid'll eat ivy, too,
Wouldn't you?"

"Hey! That was fun," Miriam said with a smile.

"Yeah," Craig said, "but that Zinney sure ain't no Pavarotti. He sounded like a wounded cow with a bad case of laryngitis. But I gotta admit, it was fun."

After clearing his throat, Zinney continued. "An exercise like this recalls something you already know; but you know it imperfectly. By refreshing your recall, you exercise the recall pathways—your recall muscles.

Recalling

"Another simple memory exercise is to read and to learn the contents of a short article in the newspaper. Once again, this might be easier by reading, writing, and reciting. However, in this exercise, it isn't important to memorize the entire article but to remember its key ideas and most important details. After you think you've learned the contents, try to recall it five or ten minutes later and again one or two hours later and then again the next day. Do the same with poems and jingles. Try to recall them a week or two later. This exercise can further secure the information in your storage bank and improve your recall pathways—your ability to retrieve information from your storage bin.

Your everyday memory

"By performing these exercises, you will improve the branching of your brain cells, increase the synapses or connections between your brain cells, and improve the overall function of your brain. You will be more knowledgeable, more confident, less forgetful, and more empowered. You'll love it."

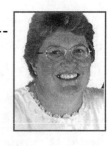

"Yeah, but will these exercises help me find my glasses or my car keys or remember the name of the guy I was just introduced to?" asked Bertha.

"Indeed they might," Zinney answered, "because they will improve your brain function. But you know there are a lot of very bright young people who have excellent brain function who habitually forget where they put their keys or glasses or even important documents. Remember, we've been forgetting things all our lives.

Remembering names

"Many of us have trouble remembering names. It's a kind of a benign absent-mindedness that results from a lack of concentration more than anything else. Forgetting names is embarrassing for many people, although it shouldn't be. One technique that I have found valuable is to repeat the person's name as you're being introduced. Look at the person as you repeat his or her name and try to identify any defining features that you might associate with that name. This may better imprint it in your memory. In the course of conversation with that person, repeat his or her name as often as possible. When you walk away from the person, mentally imagine his or her face and associate it with the name and repeat it to yourself a few times. These techniques, while not foolproof, will help.

"Sometimes nothing helps, especially when you're introduced to more than one or two people at the same time. This is clearly illustrated by the story of former President Clinton touring nursing homes. Upon entering the establishment with his entourage of special agents and reporters, he approached the elderly receptionist behind the desk and facing her eye to eye, asked, 'Pardon me, Ma'am. You know who I am, don't you?'

'No, I don't,' she responded. 'But if you go down the hall and take a left, somebody there will tell you who you are.'

The habits of remembering

"Some everyday habits that will go a long way in improving your ability to remember include organization, consistency, concentration, mental imaging, and association. The object of developing and maintaining these habits is to make it easier to remember where you put things or what tasks you have to perform on certain days. Let me explain.

"By organizing your everyday activities in a logical and consistent manner, you make it easier to remember some things. If you put your car keys in the same pocket each and every time, you are less likely to forget where you put them.

"If you place your wallet or glasses in the same place each and every time you will be less likely to misplace them. If you are inconsistent, and place these objects in different places at different times, you will have the more difficult mental task of remembering where you put them. You must develop the habit of consistency. It will work, but only if you are diligent and habitually consistent.

"It will work even better if there is some logic that can be associated with the location you've selected to place a given item. Put an insurance document or a financial document with your other insurance and financial documents. Do it as soon as you are through reviewing it or you might misplace it before you file it. If you want to look at it again for further review, you'll know exactly where to find it. A good example might be your briefcase. If you sometimes forget to bring your briefcase or some other important items to work, it might be helpful to place them in your car before retiring for the evening.

"Or, you might leave them where you would fall over them on the way to your car in the morning. At work, make your life easier. Don't allow your desk to get so cluttered that you get confused and misplace things. Handle the items on your desk one at a time and determine their importance as best you can at that time.

Frustration

"If you do misplace something, don't panic. Don't get angry with yourself. Studies have demonstrated that anger and frustration can decrease your IQ by as much as 30 points. Anger will only make it more difficult to remember and function effectively. Try to calmly rethink what you were doing when you last saw the object. Could you have covered it up with a magazine or piece of paper? Frustration and panic will only distract you by giving you something else to deal with in addition to trying to remember.

Mental imagery and association

"Each time you put something away try to use mental imagery. Try to visualize the place you put the item as you're walking away from it. In five or ten minutes, imagine yourself approaching the place where you put the item and imagine yourself retriev-

ing it. This technique is very applicable for people who forget where they parked their car. If you park your car in a large parking lot, take special care to note any landmarks surrounding the vehicle before you walk away, such as a lamppost, the entrance to a specific store, the parking level, or the number of the space. Then, as you're walking away from your car, look back at it and review these relationships. Visualize approaching your car to go home. Do this again five minutes later and again ten minutes later while you're shopping.

"This kind of disciplined association and mental imagery is often of immeasurable value in remembering. Association and mental imagery can also be of value in remembering things or tasks you want to do.

"If you have to go to the dry cleaners, the grocery, and the car wash, you can develop the mental image of the dry cleaning attendant washing your car and the grocery cashier drying it. To remember which items you need to purchase at the grocery store, write a list. You can also visualize yourself walking through the aisles of the grocery store or looking into your pantry and your refrigerator. So you see, my friends, the disciplined application of these concepts so that they become habits, can be effective in reducing some of the hassles of everyday life and make it easier for many of us.

"Once again, we're out of time. In fact we're in overtime and I know many of you want to get home."

"Wait a minute," Bertha interjected. "While we were doing those jingles, I thought of my own little rhyme I'd like to share with you, if it's okay."

"Sure," said Zinney. "Let's hear it."

"Ok! Here goes:

If our minds we recharge
our brains will enlarge.
Branching connections
will improve recollections.

So make complacency blink
while we make ourselves think.
We'll forge more synapses
and decrease relapses."

"Very good," said Zinney. "Thank you for sharing that with us, Bertha. By the way, folks, writing things like that or even trying to, is an excellent mindercise. It's good brainaerobics. Well, now we really have run out of time. I hope we all had some fun tonight. So thank you for coming and I'll look forward to seeing you next week. We'll be discussing one of your favorite topics and answering the question: Are you what you eat?"

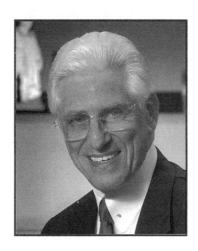

5

Your Magic Bullet

Learn the stuff
That soon will follow,
And forget the guff
That others swallow.

About 130 people were already seated in the main auditorium, which was the newly designated meeting place for Dr. Zinney's lectures. After an enthusiastic introduction by Ms. Worthington, Dr. Zinney began, "Good evening, folks. Glad you could make it here. We're gonna talk about diet and nutrition tonight. I want to encourage you to ask questions during this discussion. Remember: there are no stupid questions; there are only stupid answers, and I hope the answers I give to your questions are not any of those.

The parts of the bullet

"Most of us know that excessive body weight can be a very serious health hazard that increases the risk of developing diabetes, hypertension, heart disease, certain kinds of cancer, and a host of other maladies. Of equal significance, many of us are malnourished. That is to say, while some of us are a bit over nourished, others here appear a trifle thin; and still, some others look perfect. However, looks are deceiving and don't always reflect our state of health. There really is a magic bullet for those of you who want to lose weight and for those of you who want to gain weight. More importantly, there is a magic bullet for those who want to be healthier in the process. The magic bullet resides in a genuine understanding of nutrition and metabolism. Tonight we're going to begin our discussions on the different parts that go into making that magic bullet. They are calories, the nutrient value of food, the fiber content of our food, and dietary supplements. They are the four parts of the bullet. Recognizing that one shoe does not fit all feet and that we have different tastes and needs, each of us will have to learn to individualize the making of our bullet.

Calories

"Let's begin with the first part of the bullet, calories. Calories are the units of energy that are in the food we eat, in the proteins and fats and carbohydrates. Our bodily activities are the flames that burn these calories. Scientifically speaking, a calorie is a unit of energy that raises the temperature of one gram of water one degree Celsius. Now, proteins and carbohydrates have the same number of calories in each gram of weight. They each have four calories of energy in each gram. Fats, on the other hand, have more than twice the amount of calories in each gram of weight. Fats have nine calories in each gram. So you have to understand, it takes more than twice the amount of activity to burn the number of calories in a gram of fat than to burn the calories in a gram of carbohydrate or a gram of protein. Try to visualize a pound of fat [fig. 5A].

Not only does this pound of fat take up more space in your body than a pound of protein, it actually has more than twice as many calories than a pound of protein or a pound of carbohydrate."

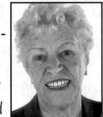

"So, Doc, that means we can eat twice as much protein or carbohydrate if we don't eat fat and still be eating the same number of calories, right?" asked Thelma.

Fat depots

"That's the right arithmetic but it's the wrong philosophy," Zinney answered. "Some fat in your diet is important. Fat produces a sense of satiety or satisfaction and certain fats are extremely important to good nutrition, the so-called Essential Fatty Acids. The important thing to remember is that the calories you eat that you don't burn by activity, can become body fat. In this regard, it makes little difference whether you get the calories from fat, carbohydrates, or proteins. If you don't burn 'em, particularly in the case of carbohydrates, they turn into body

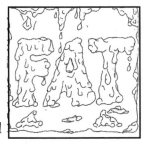

Fig 5A

60

fat. As body fat, they are a storage bank of energy. We call this storage bank *fat depots*. But sometimes, it can be as hard to get the energy out of that bank as getting a loan from First National without collateral. In order to make a withdrawal from your bank of body fat or your fat depots, you must burn more calories than you eat. When you do that, the calories that you burn in excess of the calories you eat can be withdrawn from the BOF, the bank of fat.

"This fat is distributed throughout our body but the major fat depots are in our abdomen and under our skin. In our abdomen, the fat is stored between the loops of intestines, and also behind our intestines. Excess accumulation of fat in these areas produces the classical potbelly of which we are all so fond. Excessive accumulation of fat under our skin produces generous love handles, overhanging rolls of fat in our thighs, a sagging butt and chest, a redundant neck, and flabby arms.

Calories in and calories out

"Some of you here tonight are not going to like what I have to say. But the sooner you believe it and come to grips with the facts, the sooner you will be able to help yourself. Some of you who are overweight say 'I hardly

eat anything, and I still gain weight.' Or 'I can't lose an ounce unless I starve.' I don't care what anybody tries to tell you, nobody here can gain five pounds by eating a two-pound box of chocolate. Whether you believe that or not, you must come to accept the irrefutable fact that both weight gain and weight loss is simple arithmetic: Calories In equals Calories Out. Your weight will be the result of how many calories you eat and how many calories you burn."

"Does that mean the only way I can lose weight is to count the calories I eat every day?" asked Miriam.

"No. Counting calories and grams of food is a full time job. Surely, it will help to have a reasonable idea of how many calories are in the food we eat and how many calories we burn during the day. In this regard, a good nutritionist, calorie charts, weight reducing parlors and recipe books can be of value in helping to guide you to your individual goal; but with or without this assistance, you must be in control. The truth that sets you free is when you get on the scale and you count your pounds, not your calories.

More importantly, our interest should be focused on good nutrition and body composition, our percentage of body fat relative to our muscle mass. We'll discuss this in some detail a little later.

"For those of us who should reduce, it must be acknowledged that some people can lose weight more easily than others. Eating habits, exercise habits and dedication are important; but it isn't just a matter of will power. Genetically determined differences in intestinal function, tastes and metabolism play important roles. So let's discuss some of these things now.

Burn, build, or blubber

"Proteins, carbohydrates, and fats are metabolized through different but intimately inter-related pathways. The proteins we eat are broken down and are absorbed as amino acids. These are the building blocks of tissue protein, of muscle [fig. 5B]. The fat that we eat is absorbed as glycerol, fatty acids and triglycerides, or just plain fat. The carbohydrates you eat are converted to simple sugars. They, in turn, are converted to glucose, the simple sugar that circulates in our blood [fig. 5C].

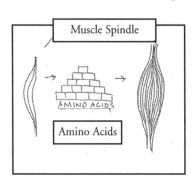

Fig 5B

"This takes place through the digestive process in our intestines and through the metabolic pathway for carbohydrates.

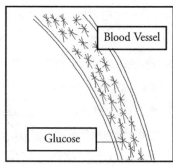

Fig 5

"This sugar, glucose, is our source of immediate energy. The glucose that is not used for immediate energy is stored in our liver and in our muscles in the form of a starch called glycogen [fig. 5D].

"This starch, glycogen, is a source of stored energy for our muscles. However, if the glycogen

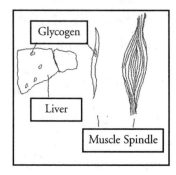

Fig

in our muscles and liver is not used for energy, it too can be converted to fat and find a comfy resting-place in our fat depots. As we said, the glucose in our blood that is not quickly burned for energy must find a storage place in muscle or liver glycogen. If these storage capacities are filled, it can be converted to fat and also join its cousins in a comfy fat depot. So excess carbohydrate calories that are not used for energy are converted to fat and excess protein calories that are not used for tissue and muscle building or for energy are converted to fat [fig. 5E].

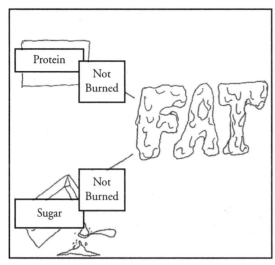

Fig 5E

"In different individuals, some metabolic pathways are or may become more firmly established than others. So some people may have a greater percentage of the calories they eat converted to fat and others may have a greater percentage of the calories they eat converted to building muscle. The varying efficiency of these metabolic pathways may be determined, in part, by repeated use of these pathways; however, they may also be determined, in part, by our genetic make up. Individuals who eat a large number of calories each day, particularly in the form of carbohydrates; and don't burn them through activity, store these calories as fat. In this way, the metabolic pathway for converting calories to fat becomes increasingly efficient and the metabolic pathways for burning energy and building muscle become progressively inefficient. On the other hand, people who exercise and increase their metabolic rate may develop more efficient pathways to burn calories and build muscle.

"It's conceivable that the same is true for the mechanisms of intestinal absorption. People who acclimate to a high fiber diet tolerate it satisfactorily and are not troubled by excess gaseousness. It's conceivable that people who eat a high fat diet develop the digestive process for fats more effectively so that fats are more easily absorbed and stored in their fat depots. Still, when the rubber hits the road, it's Calories In and Calories Out.

The insulin effect

"Remember, when you eat carbohydrates it becomes blood glucose. This rise in your blood sugar level stimulates your pancreas to produce insulin to process the glucose. This has been called the glycemic effect of food. As you might have guessed, carbohydrates, like sugars and starches, have the strongest insulin or glycemic effect. The glucose will then be burned as energy or converted to glycogen or to fat by the action of insulin. The chronic overeating of carbohydrates, particularly sugars, can then cause a chronic rise in your insulin level. This can result in the production of more and more fat. Many people who have been overweight for several years are victims of this vicious circle of events. Perhaps there is a genetic proclivity for this; but surely, carbohydrate overindulgence is the major culprit. While restriction of carbohydrate intake in these individuals is very important, it is also important to re-establish the efficiency of the metabolic pathways used to build muscle and utilize energy."

The genetic effect

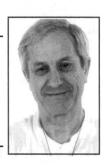

"Dr. Zinney, Sam here. I know people where everyone in the whole family is fat. Is this some kind of hereditary thing?"

"We all know overweight people whose whole family is obese. In some cases, this may be due to poor eating and exercise habits that are passed on from one generation to the next. However, we have much more to learn about the role played by genes and hormones in the distribution of body fat and the development of obesity. A genetic determinant regarding the efficiency of different metabolic pathways and absorptive abilities of the intestinal tract for carbohydrates, fats, and proteins or even a genetic proclivity to enjoy the taste of certain fattening foods might be important.

"A better understanding of some of these issues has been further effaced by the recent discovery of the *ob* gene and the newly appreciated actions of certain hormones. The *ob* gene governs the production of a hormone, called *leptin*. This hormone appears to be produced by our fat cells and its activity serves to reduce body fat. On the flip side, the stomach produces a different hormone called *ghrelin*. This hormone increases appetite and food intake. It also decreases the metabolic rate and the breakdown of body fat. An increase or decrease in the productivity or activity of these hormones might be, at least in part, genetically determined. Conceivably, all of these factors and more that are yet to be unveiled could interact to make weight control more difficult for some than for others.

"An example that makes the same point may be seen in the case of two bodybuilders each eating the same diet and each working out equally as hard. One may develop an excellent and very healthy body and the other may become a Mr. Universe. The metabolic pathways for burning energy and building muscle may have been more efficient in Mr. Universe by reason of his genetic make up. While its important to appreciate all of this, none of it alters the validity of the concept of Calories In and Calories Out.

Myths

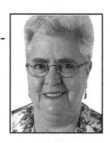
"There are people with heart, kidney, or liver disease who do indeed suffer from water retention. Also, there are some medications that people take that can result in water retention, another cause of weight gain. We call this edema. If you think you are retaining water, then you should consult your physician to see if you have any of these problems. On other occasions, people can have a meal or two containing an enormous amount of salt and experience transient water retention; but this usually disappears in a day or two. Most people who say they're overweight because of water retention only avoid dealing with the problem.

"There are several other misconceptions that may hold us back from losing weight. There are those of us who believe that we weigh more because we have 'big bones.' That's another myth. Trust me, a five-year old child could lift your entire skeleton with one hand.

"Some of us eat more than we admit; and many of us eat more than we realize.

Basal or resting metabolic rate (RMR)

"The rate at which we burn calories at rest is called the Resting Metabolic Rate or RMR. Calories burned at rest, even when we're sleeping, provide the energy to maintain our bodily functions—to keep us breathing, to keep our heart beating, to keep our intestinal tract functioning and the like. Recently, a handheld device, called BodyGem™, has been developed that can determine your RMR by having you breathe into it for several minutes. Alternatively, you can estimate your RMR by multiplying your weight by ten. For example: if you weigh 150 pounds, your RMR is approximately 1500 calories a day. However, this is only a *guesstimate* of your RMR because a pound of muscle burns 40-50 calories a day AT REST; and a pound of fat only burns 2 calories a day. So, two people weighing exactly the same but having a different body composition may have vastly different RMR expenditures. Those of us with a lower percent of body fat and a greater percent of muscle mass will burn far more calories even at rest. This could amount to more than a thousand calories a day, emphasizing the importance of adding muscle mass while losing weight."

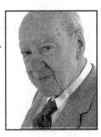

A well-dressed gentleman from the audience interrupted, "But Dr. Zinney, don't some people just naturally burn more calories than others?"

"To some extent you're right. Some of it is related to the genetic issues and the metabolic pathways we've discussed but most of it is related to our body composition and our activity. Our resting metabolic rate continues throughout the day; but when we are more active, we utilize more energy and burn even more calories. So you see, the total number of calories we burn equals the number of calories burned as a result of our RMR and the calories we burn as a result of activity—standing, walking, climbing stairs, exercising and the like. If we are sedentary throughout the day, we might add 20% to 40% to our RMR caloric expenditure to determine our total daily caloric burn. If we are moderately active or very active, this might be increased by 50% to 80% a day or even higher as a result of a regular exercise program. Remember—the more muscle and less fat you have in your body the more calories you burn, even at rest. Your RMR is higher. Also, having more muscle and less fat enables you to increase your daily activity and burn even more calories even more efficiently.

"That said, if you burn more calories than you eat, you will lose weight. If you eat more calories than you burn, you will gain weight. It's that simple—Calories In and Calories Out.

Age and glandular conditions

"This is one reason the basal metabolic rate of burning calories decreases with age. As we age, our muscle mass decreases, our activity decreases, and the basal metabolic rate decreases. At the age of seventy, most of us have a decrease in basal metabolic rate of about ten percent. Clearly, this could result in weight gain.

"Other conditions, such as a thyroid hormone deficiency, can decrease the basal metabolic rate and cause weight gain. This can usually be treated rather easily with thyroid hormone. But that's beyond the scope of this discussion. On the other hand, the basal metabolic rate can be increased by stress, by illness, by an overactive thyroid, and even by fever. In elderly people, in particular, this can result in weight loss, malnutrition, and dehydration.

"Add to this that many older folks have poor dental structures and many have developed poor dietary habits for several decades. Some are also taking medications that change their appetite. All of this can create malnutrition, further endangering survival.

However, when you consider everything, it still comes down to Calories In and Calories Out. In this way, you are what you eat. You are what you eat, what you know, what you do, what you've done, and what you can do. That's what you are."

Craig whispered to his niece Bertha who was raising her hand, "If we are what we eat, let's go out and eat something very, very rich."

Depression and your weight

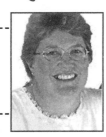

"Dr. Zinney," Bertha asked, "what effect does depression have?"

"Many people eat because they're depressed. It can be a way of rewarding themselves, of making them feel more comfortable. Depressive disorders can result in obesity. In other instances, depression can dampen the appetite and cause severe weight loss and malnutrition.

Body fat

"We now know that the more muscle mass we have in our body in relation to our body fat, the more calories we burn, even at rest. Also, increasing our muscle strength and endurance will enable us to enjoy activities that will burn still more calories. For example, three pounds of muscle could burn as much as 9,000 calories a month. So adding three pounds of muscle means that you could lose about thirty pounds a year without even changing your diet.

"But body fat is important! We all need it. It helps us regulate our body temperature; it serves as a storage depot of energy; it cushions our joints and protects our vital organs; it stores vitamins and it's used to make hormones. So some fat in our diets, particularly those that contain the so-called essential fatty acids, is vital to good health. What we don't need is too much body fat. An excess of body fat is associated with diabetes, high cholesterol, heart disease, hypertension, cancer, and God only knows what other not-so-nice things. Within reasonable parameters, achieving the proper ratio of body fat to muscle, is more important than achieving our ideal weight.

Ideal weight

"We'll discuss how to measure your body fat a little later, but first let's talk about what is meant by ideal weight," said Zinney. "These are categories based on height, age, and gender as shown in this slide [fig. 5F]."

Audible gasps came from the audience as they studied the slide. "My God," said someone. "If I weighed that little, I'd be a scarecrow."

Height (feet, inches)	Weight Ranges (in pounds)			
	Minimum for all adults (BMI=20)	Recommended maximum for ages up to 25 years	Recommended maximum for ages between 25 & 45 years	Maximum for all Adults (45+) (BMI=25)
4'9"	92	106	111	115
4'10"	95	110	115	119
4'11"	99	114	119	124
5'0"	102	118	123	128
5'1"	106	121	127	132
5'2"	109	125	131	136
5'3"	113	130	135	141
5'4"	116	134	140	145
5'5"	120	138	144	150
5'6"	124	142	148	155
5'7"	127	147	153	159
5'8"	131	151	158	164
5'9"	135	155	162	169
5'10"	139	160	167	174
5'11"	143	165	172	179
6'0"	147	169	177	184
6'1"	151	174	182	189
6'2"	155	179	187	194
6'3"	160	184	192	200
6'4"	164	189	197	205

Fig 5F

Zinney continued, "While useful in a general sense, they were probably popularized by insurance actuarial departments and have been based on the fact that obesity can compromise longevity. It's important to note, however, that people who are less than twenty percent over their ideal weight have no significant increased risk in regard to longevity."

"Doc, I'm not sure I understand what you mean," said Kinder.

"I'll explain," Zinney said. "The chart of ideal weight is adjusted for height, gender, and age and can serve as one of the guidelines for good health. However, if you weigh less than twenty percent more than your ideal weight, your risk of death or disease is not significantly greater than someone who is at their ideal weight.

Measuring body composition by BMI

"As I've said, what is really important to your health is your muscle-to-fat ratio. This is far more important than the ideal weights listed on some insurance company charts. One of the most widely used methods of estimating body composition is the Body Mass Index, often referred to as the BMI.

"For those of you who like mathematics, calculating your BMI is a good way to get an understanding of your body composition, and whether or not you should be classified as obese or otherwise at increased risk for cardiovascular complications. You can do it with pencil and paper; but it's much easier if you have a calculator, especially if you're as bad at math as I am. If you can measure your height and weight yourself using the metric system, it's much easier. If you can't, then you have to convert inches to meters and pounds to kilograms. The formula to calculate your BMI is simple. Divide your weight in kilograms by the square of your height in meters [kg/m^2].

"George A. Bray, M.D. has simplified this by developing a nomogram [see pg. 74] that allows you to determine your BMI in three easy steps. Note that the chart has three columns. Body weight, in pounds and kilograms, is in the column

68

on the left. Height, in inches and centimeters, is in the column on the right, and the BMI is in the middle column. First identify your weight in pounds or kilograms and put a straight edge, or ruler, across the chart at that level. Second, identify your height in inches or in centimeters and put another straight edge, or ruler, across the chart at that level. Your BMI can be found in the middle column at the midpoint between the two straight edges or rulers.

"While those of us with a BMI greater than 30 are classified as obese, the risk of cardiovascular disease progressively increases at BMI levels above twenty-five. Recognizing this, I believe all of us should strive to have a BMI of 25 or less. If your BMI is higher, you're probably eating too many drippy grilled cheese sandwiches and not getting enough exercise.

Other ways of measuring body fat

"The most accurate method of determining your percentage of body fat requires the use of a DEXA scan or an elaborate device that weighs you in a cold water bath. The latter may be available in some fitness centers. There are also calipers that measure your fat content by pinching your skin and fat at different locations. I call them 'pinch-an-inch' devices and have no confidence in their accuracy. However, the distribution of body fat does appear to have substantial implica-

tions in regard to obesity related morbidity. Many of the more important complications of obesity are linked to upper body fat. Specifically, intra-abdominal obesity and abdominal wall fat (the potbelly) are associated with a greater frequency of cardiovascular complications than lower body fat—fat buttocks and thighs.

"The distinction can be easily made by measuring your waist and your hips with a tape measure. A waist to hip ratio of greater than 0.9 in females and 1.0 in males is indicative of excessive upper abdominal fat and a further increase in the risk of obesity related morbidity. Here again, consistency is important. Keep in mind that fluctuations in abdominal gaseous distension, the levels at which you apply the tape measure, and the amount of tension you apply to it can affect the accuracy of these measurements.

"For those of you who want an easy way to measure your body fat, there are several affordable handheld devices on the market that are reasonably accurate. They work through infra-red technology and can be purchased at most sporting goods stores. There are even bathroom scales on the market that will tell your weight and your percent of body fat, which work through bio-electric technology. While not as accurate as a DEXA scan or cold water bath scale, they're a convenient way of establishing a base line and monitoring your progress.

"It isn't essential that you use one of these devices. If you eat a healthful diet, monitor your weight, and get the proper exercise, you will decrease your body fat, increase your muscle mass, and take inches off in all the right places. If you can, however, I urge you to splurge and buy one of these convenient devices to get a better idea of your percent of body fat. Decreasing your percentage of body fat while approaching your ideal weight is much more important than simply achieving your ideal weight."

"What should it be?" asked Bertha. "What's the right percentage of body fat we should have?"

"The answer to that is variable," Zinney answered. "It varies with gender and age and also who you believe. Many professional athletes and bodybuilders maintain body fat levels of five to fifteen percent. That's a lot lower than I'm suggesting for most of us. Our livelihoods aren't dependent on our athletic performance. In my opinion, adult women should ideally have a body fat content that ranges between twenty-three to thirty-five percent and men, between fifteen to twenty percent or even up to twenty five percent after

sixty. The chart I'm projecting on the screen shows the proper range of body fat percentage for males and females in different age groups [fig. 5G].

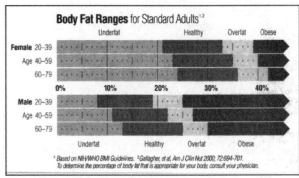

Chart printed with permission from Tanita Corporation of America, Inc.

Fig 5G

Counting calories or counting pounds

"While we might recommend that the average-sized adult male eat 2500 calories a day and the average female eat 2000 calories a day, these recommendations can't apply to everyone. That could be perfect for the person who burns 2500 or 2000 calories a day and who has a body fat content in the range of twenty percent. If you burn more calories, you can eat more calories to maintain your body weight and your fat ratio.

"Some professional athletes, as result of their workouts and sports activities, eat more than 5000 calories a day to maintain their body weight and fat ratio. But if your body weight and fat ratio is higher than it should be, then you have to eat less and burn more by increasing your activity and your exercise."

"Well, is that it? We eat what we like and then exercise till we drop. Don't we have to weigh our food or count all the calories in what we eat?" asked Bertha.

"The answer is no, no, and no again," Zinney responded. "I don't want anybody to exercise until they drop. Eating sensibly and exercising sensibly will have the cumulative effect of improving the metabolic pathways that build muscle and burn energy more efficiently. As this develops, you will build more muscle mass, have more energy, and improve your health.
Your percentage of body fat will decrease and your vigor and strength will increase.

"Think about this: if you eat just a mere 100 calories a day more than you burn each day, you can gain as much as 10 pounds in a year. Within reason, you don't have to count calories but you do have to weigh yourself. That's where the rubber hits the road. If you weigh more today than you weighed yesterday then you ate more calories yesterday than you burned. If you want to lose weight, you must take a corrective action and burn more calories today than you eat today. If you want to gain weight then you must eat more calories than you burn. You don't have to sit in a corner every day and plot your menus down to the last calorie. You can learn to increase lean muscle weight and lose that extra fat.

"Actually, calories are your friends, not your enemies. A general idea of the calories you eat is important. But actually counting the calories and grams of every thing you eat is so difficult for most people that it causes them to fail.

"Let's take a look at how someone might decide how many calories you should eat: A well-intentioned dietician or nutritionist decides you're overweight and puts you on a 1700 calorie diet.

"If you're burning 1600 calories a day, you won't lose weight. You'll gain weight. Remember what we said, if you eat 100 calories each day more than you burn, you can gain ten pounds a year. If you're on a 3000 calorie diet and you burn 4000 calories a day, you will lose weight. So, determining the amount of calories you should eat is purely a *guesstimate* that guesses or estimates how many calories you will burn. That's exactly what I want you to do—estimate the calories you take in and estimate the calories you burn. Your guess will become increasingly accurate and fine-tuned by weighing yourself each day.

"Sure, I know that some psychologists and dieticians say you shouldn't weigh yourself every day because you'll get discouraged and depressed if you haven't lost weight; and then you might abandon their calorie counting program. But then you don't know what's working and what's not. That's the ostrich syndrome: You bury your head in the sand so you don't know what's working and what's not. Then, ten days later you find out that you've gained five pounds by counting the calories wrong or counting the wrong calories.

"If you're trying to lose weight and you weigh more today than you weighed yesterday, then you ate more calories than you burned and corrective action should be taken."

"What kind of corrective action do you mean?" asked Bertha.

"You have to eat less and burn more. The effect may be immediate or it may take a few days, but it will happen for you. It may mean that you have to add an extra ten minutes to your walking or your workout schedule for a few days. And you may have to decrease the size of your portions, but it will happen. You'll lose it. Every day is a new experience. You're in control," Zinney answered.

Calories vs. exercise

"But which is more important," Bertha asked, "increasing my exercise or decreasing what I eat?"

"They're both important. If you ask me

which one has a quicker effect on weight loss, the answer is eating less. For example, there are about 3500 calories in a pound of fat. A one-mile walk will burn about 100 calories. So theoretically, you would have to walk 35 miles to lose a pound of fat. If you view this in a narrow sense, you'd have to wonder why you should exercise at all. What's the point? On the other hand if you ate 200 calories less and burned 150 calories more, you would lose a pound of fat every ten days. If you ate 500 calories less and burned an extra 500 calories a day, you would lose two pounds of fat each week.

"Exercise is important for many reasons. If you lose weight without adding muscle, you may weigh less; but you might not be much healthier. Studies have actually shown that obese men who are physically fit have greater longevity than normal weight men who are not physically fit. This doesn't mean that being obese is good. Obesity has many health risks. However, the study does underscore the value of exercise and physical fitness. Some of the weight loss, especially in cases of very rapid weight loss, may be the loss of muscle mass as well as fat. As we discussed previously, muscle tissue burns more calories than fat tissue—even at rest. So, a far healthier and more effective program is to balance calorie eating with calorie burning by exercise and building muscle. This approach has a far more beneficial effect on your percentage of body fat. As your muscle mass increases, you will be able to eat more calories. Actually, you may need more calories to stay in balance. But, remember, animal studies have suggested that caloric restriction can increase longevity. So the object of eating just enough to build lean muscle and improve physical performance is the ideal balance.

"We'll really get into talking about exercise in the next few weeks, so you be sure to stick around, folks."

Weigh yourself everyday

"Dr. Zinney, I used to weigh myself everyday and found crazy changes in my weight that could never be explained by what you said. How do you explain that?" asked Miriam.

"Daily weight may fluctuate for quite some time until your caloric expenditure and your newly-improved metabolic pathways have been conditioned. After that, daily weighing will become increasingly valuable as a guide to your performance. Take note, however, it will be important for you to have a good scale and to weigh yourself the same time of day, each and every day, without clothing, and after or before your morning toilet. Consistency is most important. Most bathroom scales are spring scales. If you are using a spring scale, your posture and the position of your feet on the scale can affect the reading by as much as

three or more pounds. Be certain that the position of your feet and your posture are the same from day to day. Remember, consistency is important.

Menus and recipes

"In terms of specific menus, there are numerous diet books, recipe books, cooking books, and menu lists available. They have been around for years and haven't been successful in producing a healthy population. Some of them are full of helpful ideas, but all of them are useless unless you have some appreciation of nutrition and your own metabolism. If you do, these diet and recipe books can be of service. Understanding how metabolism, genetics, eating habits, and exercise habits interact will enable us to better apply the simple concept of Calories In and Calories Out.

"Next week we'll discuss more about the three major food categories: proteins, carbohydrates, and fats. We will also learn about fiber, minerals, and vitamins. We must learn what they are, where they are, and what they can do **for** or **to** us. We must learn how much of each can help us achieve the goal we set for ourselves and what foods have the highest quality of these nutrients. Then we can learn how to develop the self-customized program and diet that we, as individuals, can enjoy. That's our topic for next week. Thank you for coming tonight and I'll look forward to seeing all of you again."

Body Mass Index

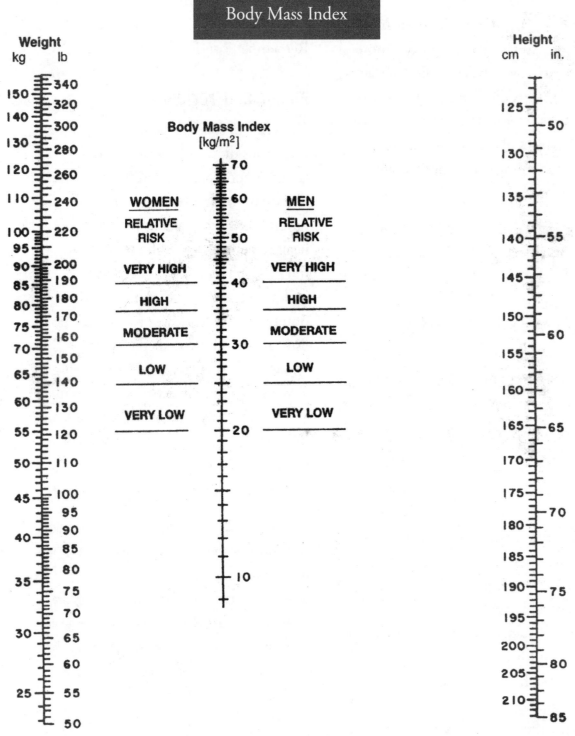

Nomogram for determining body mass index. To use this nomogram, place a ruler or other straight edge between the body weight (without clothes) in kilograms or pounds located on the left-hand line and the height (without shoes) in centimeters or in inches located on the right-hand line. The body mass index is read from the middle of the scale and is in metric units. (*Copyright 1978, George A. Bray, MD. Used with permission.*)

74

6

Breathe clean air,
Eat good greens,
If you care —
Here's the means.

Groans,
Grumbles,
and Gases

As people were filing into the auditorium, Martha Worthington and Zinney conversed casually at the podium. "That was a complicated subject you discussed last week," said Martha.

Fad diets

"Well, Martha," Zinney replied, "metabolism is indeed a complicated topic. A lot of weight reduction programs manipulate metabolic pathways to get short-term weight loss. Some of them rely on strict abstinence from carbohydrates and the development of ketosis to burn fat and others rely too heavily on negative will power. Fat burning diets, crash starvation diets, or fad diets can cause very rapid weight loss but that doesn't necessarily make you healthier.

"As I've said, many of these programs don't place enough emphasis on body composition—the importance of decreasing your percentage of body fat and increasing your percentage of lean muscle mass through exercise. In fact, if you lose weight too rapidly, you lose valuable muscle mass, not just fat. For most people who have to lose 75 pounds or less, I recommend that they do it slowly—about one to three pounds a week. Losing it more rapidly is very likely to result in a loss of important muscle mass. There's a little rhyme called the Chunky Blues that sort of sums it up. It goes something like this:

You might have the Chunky-Blues
From some extra pounds you can't excuse.
But as you muse the Don'ts and Do's
Here's some views you might peruse:

Avoid that fad and its hyped-up ruse
And the metabolic myth it spews.
Crashy diets make big news,
But be aware of the guile they use.

Those flashy ads that light your fuse,
With the pills and breakthroughs
they enthuse,
Are just the claims we should recuse;
Cause it's our health they could
abuse.

Check your diet's P's and Q's
And the fact or fiction it accrues.
You're in charge of what ensues
And you can drop the weight you
choose.

So don't refuse to take these clues—
It's not a race; it's a healthful cruise.
Shed those pounds in ones and twos
And you will lose the Chunky-Blues.

"And while some people are very disciplined and can follow a healthful diet forever, most of us find it very difficult. Asking people to deny themselves anything they think they really want will usually set them up to fail. It's my belief that people are better equipped to make important modifications in their lifestyle if they understand the reasons why those modifications are important. It's the key to the simple concept of Calories In and Calories Out."

Fat substitutes and carbohydrates

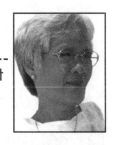

"I think you did a good job, but you really made carbohydrates out to be bad guys. Is that really true?" Martha asked.

"I didn't think I did that. At least I didn't mean to do that; and I'm glad you're calling it to my attention," said Zinney. "Carbs can be bad guys if you eat the low fiber carbs and not enough of the high fiber carbs. The low fiber carbs are quickly converted to sugar and if you don't burn them, they turn to fat. Actually, it's one of the reasons a lot of low-fat substitutes have failed to help people lose weight."

"What do you mean?" asked Martha.

"Many people eat low-fat or no-fat substitute snacks that are loaded with low fiber carbs. Because they're low in fat and sometimes low in fiber, they're not as satisfying or filling. So people tend to overeat them. Those carbs turn to sugar and then to fat. Among other important health benefits, high fiber carbs are filling. They are also an abundant source of very important nutrients, vitamins, and antioxidants. I'll make sure to clarify these differences tonight."

After a quick introduction by Ms. Worthington, Dr. Zinney took the microphone and began, "Good evening, ladies and gentlemen, and welcome. For those of you who are new here tonight, I'm Dr. Zinney. Last week we discussed metabolism and tonight we will carry the discussion further into the realm of nutrition. We will examine the role that proteins, carbohydrates, fats, fiber, and dietary supplements might play in our lives; and each of us will attempt to determine what's best for us as individuals.

"Probably, many of us have a long history of bad dietary habits and we may have to make some changes in our diet. I'm not going to suggest that you follow a specific dietary prescription or some new fad diet. Many of them work well for a time and many of them have long-term drawbacks. Most of them are based on the belief that you won't exercise in order to burn more calories and build more muscle. Others seem to be based on the principle that if tastes good, you should spit it out. If you really want to win in the second half, you WILL definitely have to exercise. And it is likely that you will have to change some of your eating habits. But whatever changes might be necessary, your nutritional intake must be in keeping with your individual tastes or you won't stick

with them.

"Some modifications may be more difficult for some than for others; but keep in mind that your tastes have changed over the years. You may find some new changes quite enjoyable after you try them for a while. Many of us know people who have given up red meat for a period of time; and then, when attempting to eat it, find it disagreeable. While all of us know that change for the better is desirable; change, of any kind, is commonly viewed as difficult. The objective of tonight's discussion will be to keep the groans and grumbles from becoming screams by having you learn how to make modifications that are acceptable to you. You will learn how to fashion your own nutritional program.

Positive commitment and the pleasures of eating

"For most of us, eating is one of the many great pleasures in life and I believe it should stay that way. The use of will power to avoid eating certain foods, foods that we really enjoy, has not proven effective in changing bad eating habits. This is because we are attempting to use will power in a negative way. Negative will power says don't eat this and don't eat that.

"The kind of power that we should use is *the power of positive commitment.* It should be directed at what we should eat—not what we shouldn't eat. Let's take the guy who likes to eat two or three doughnuts with coffee every morning. Instead of telling himself that he can't eat those doughnuts, he now tells himself that he can. But first, he must eat a high fiber cereal or an egg-white omelet with high fiber vegetables, some whole-wheat toast, and a glass of skim milk. After that breakfast, if he still wants a doughnut, it's his. Instead of eating two or three doughnuts, he may eat one, or one half, or a bite, or none. The nutritious and filling breakfast that he satisfied him. The decision he made was not to avoid doughnuts; it was to eat something good for him, to eat the right foods."

"But, Doc, I can't eat breakfast," Sam exclaimed. "It makes me nauseous. I haven't eaten breakfast in more than twenty years."

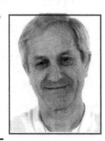

"That's what you made yourself believe. That's only a habit. You're denying your body a very important metabolic kick in the morning because of a bad habit that you developed. Most people who have this habit actually know how good breakfast is for them. Recall your childhood. Your mother made sure you had a nutritious breakfast before you left for school? Chances are, you did that for your children, too.

"Look at it this way, Sam, I'm not suggesting that you deny yourself a darn thing. I'm suggesting that you do something that you're not doing now—eat enough of something good. To the extent that you believe that this requires some commitment on your part, I agree with you. That's the commitment I want you to make, to do something good for yourself that you're not doing now.

"This approach is just as applicable to the burger, hot dog, or pizza addict at lunch or dinner. It may be perceived by some of you as an oversimplification but it isn't. It's real. It's a change in paradigm or viewpoint and it works. Use your will power to eat something that's good for you, and you won't have to use your will power to avoid that piece of apple pie or coconut cream pie. If you eat enough of the right foods in a balanced diet, and you still want that piece of pie, then have at it. But here again, you may find that you want a smaller piece of pie or just a bite or none at all. Your knowledge that the pie is full of fat and low fiber carbohydrates that

78

will be converted to fat, combined with your sense of fullness from eating something that's good for you, may change your level of desire. What you must be sure to do is to eat enough of the good stuff. Don't train yourself to leave room for the pie."

The balanced diet

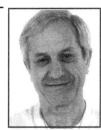

"Hey, Doc!" exclaimed Sam. "I never thought of it that way. You're right! I think I can do it. But, Doc, help us out. Tell us what a balanced diet is, or at least what you mean by a balanced diet."

"Good question, Sam. The United States Department of Agriculture developed a food pyramid to serve as guidelines for a balance diet. I'll project it on the screen for us [fig. 6A]. They're supposed to update this every five years but have delayed doing so because of controversy. Most authorities believe that these guidelines are too high in sugars, starches, grains, fats and red meat. The pyramid might have been a bad idea to begin with but its gotten an even worse rap than it deserves. Many blame this faulty pyramid for contributing to the growing obesity of America, but I don't know too many fat people who have

ever even looked at it. Here are some of the important changes I believe should be made: stay low on the fat, sugars and starches. Also, use fish and poultry as a major source of protein instead of red meat.

"Now, everyone talks about a serving of this and a serving of that; but it's been brought to my attention that most of us don't really know what it is that constitutes a serving. So let me address that first; and then, we'll discuss the various food categories. At the end of this evening, I'll summarize my view of a healthful balanced diet. You might call it *Zinney's Zummary*.

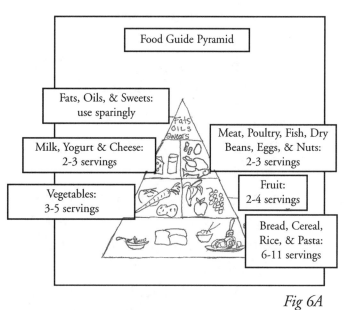

Fig 6A

What is "a serving"?

"Here's a list that will give you a good idea of how much food makes up a serving in each of the food categories.

Grains

1 slice of bread
1/2 cup of cooked rice or pasta
1/2 cup of cooked cereal
1 ounce of ready-to-eat cereal

Fruits

1 piece of fruit
1 melon wedge
3/4 cup of fruit juice
1/2 cup canned fruit
1/4 cup dried fruit

Vegetables

1/2 cup of chopped raw or cooked vegetables
1 cup of leafy raw vegetables

Milk, Yogurt, and Cheese

1 cup of milk or yogurt
1-1/2 to two ounces of cheese
Example: a 1-inch cube of hard cheese weighs about 1/2 ounce

Notes:
Buy low-fat or skim dairy products to avoid harmful fats.
Some people have trouble digesting lactose, the sugar in milk products. If you have this problem, try eating yogurt with active cultures, low-fat cheese, or lactose reduced milk. Pills and drops that help digest lactose are also available.

Meat, Poultry, Fish, Dry Beans, Eggs and Nuts

1/2 cup of cooked beans, 1 egg or 2 tablespoons of peanut butter make up 1/3 of a serving of this food group.

2- 1/2 to 3 ounces of cooked lean meat poultry or fish make up one serving of this food group.

Examples: a slice of cooked, lean meat or poultry that is about 1/4- inch thick and measures 3 inches by 4 inches weighs about 2 ounces; a cooked lean hamburger patty that weighs 3 ounces is about 3 inches across and 1/2- inch thick - about the size of a large mayonnaise jar lid.

Note: Before cooking, a patty this size weighs 4 ounces.

Note: Half of a skinless, cooked chicken breast weighs about 3 ounces.

Note: Egg whites are a good source of protein, but egg yolks are high in fat and cholesterol. Consider discarding the yolk.

Note: Nuts are a source of protein and antioxidants but are high in calories.

Note: Limit your intake of sugar, sweets and red meat.

"Again, we're not going to get into recipes or menus. There are plenty of books that can be helpful in this regard if you think you need them. Try to balance your tastes with a diet that is abundant in high fiber carbohydrates and protein and low in sugars, starches and the fats derived from red meat or poultry skin. High fiber carbs and proteins keep you full. They produce a sense of satiety. They keep you satisfied longer.

"Proteins are absorbed more slowly than starches and sugars and provide a more steady flow of energy instead of the roller coaster swings that occur with eating sugars. You know, you eat starches or sugars and your blood sugar goes up and then the insulin secretion goes up to manage the surge in blood glucose. When the surge in blood glucose is brought down by the insulin surge, you eat more starches or sugar. That's the roller coaster effect— up and down, and up and down again. It's a vicious circle that can be avoided by eating protein and high fiber carbohydrates.

Proteins

"Let's begin with proteins. You will recall that there are four calories of energy in each gram of protein. Proteins are made of amino acids, which are the building blocks of our tissue protein. When we eat protein, our digestive tract breaks them down into amino acids for absorption. After these amino acids are absorbed, they are reconstituted into tissue protein to service our individual needs. This is the stuff that makes up our muscles— the muscle tissue in our arms, legs,

and the tissue in our faces that enable us to smile and frown. This is the stuff that makes the muscles in our mouths and throats that enable us to swallow and to speak. All of these are the somatic muscles—the muscles that make up the musculo-skeletal system."

"I don't have to worry much about speaking," Craig whispered to Sam. "I haven't talked to my wife in three weeks."

"Why? Are you guys having a problem?" asked Sam.

"No! I just don't want to interrupt her," quipped Craig.

Zinney continued, "The muscle tissue in our blood vessels and heart pump and circulate the blood throughout our body. The muscle tissue in our esophagus and intestinal tract propel our food and nutrients for the purpose of digestion and excretion. These are the muscles of our viscera and they too are made up of tissue protein. And so, you can grasp the importance of this protein stuff.

"There are complete proteins and incomplete proteins. Complete proteins are proteins that contain all of the essential amino acids; and incomplete proteins are proteins that contain some, but not all, of the essential amino acids. There are eight essential amino acids. These are the amino acids that our scientists have found to be necessary for building healthy tissue. Their chemical names might not be important for you to remember but I'll tell you what they are anyway: leucine, isoleucine, methionine, valine, phenylalanine, lysine, tryptophan, and threonine. If you're going to take a protein supplement, having a list of these might help you determine the quality of the supplement. Oh yeah, histadine is a ninth one for children because it's so important for growth and development. Eggs, particularly egg-white, and milk and animal protein are the best sources of these high quality complete proteins. The proteins in most vegetables are incomplete proteins because they don't contain all of the essential amino acids. So if you're a vegetarian and you want to get your proteins from vegetables, you must have a mixed and varied diet of vegetables to be sure of getting all the essential amino acids."

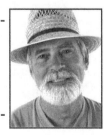

"Doc! John Kinder here again! About how much protein should we get a day?"

"John, you must be a clairvoyant," Zinney responded. "That's just the subject I was about to address. The recommended daily intake of protein varies with age, gender, and muscle mass. For example, protein require-

ments are higher during adolescence than during adulthood and higher during pregnancy and lactation. People with a large muscle mass or who are exercising and building muscle need more protein than people with a smaller amount of muscle mass.

"Taking all this into consideration, many authorities believe the average adult should eat forty-five to sixty-five grams of protein a day. Others feel that thirty percent of your total daily caloric intake should be in the form of protein. For example, if you are eating a 2,000 calorie diet, six hundred calories could be consumed in the form of protein rich foods (fish, chicken, turkey, etc.). Since there are four calories in each gram of protein, that might amount to about 150 grams a day. If you are a more heavily muscled person, or if you are on a muscle building exercise program, you may require more than that amount. However, many are concerned about a diet that is too high in protein, particularly in individuals with kidney or liver problems. While too much protein can sometimes be hard for these organs to handle, I believe the dangers of this in normal people have been over-exaggerated. Most people with normally functioning kidneys and a normal liver can handle the recommended amounts of protein without any difficulty. People with kidney disease or advanced liver disease and people with risk factors for kidney disease such as heart disease, hypertension or diabetes should check with their doctor to determine how much protein is appropriate for them.

"There are some additional notes of caution. You must eat a balanced diet of protein, carbohydrate, and some fat. If the proportion of your daily calories is too high in protein and too low in carbohydrate, you won't be able to utilize all that protein for building tissue protein. Some will be stored as fat or glycogen, or the body will try to use it for energy by converting the protein into sugar, but it's not an efficient source of ready energy.

"Also, if you eat too many calories at one time, even in the form of lean healthy protein, you will store the excess calories that you don't use or burn as glycogen or fat. That's one problem some people experience who eat one meal a day or who eat most of their total daily calories at one meal. It's a very good reason to distribute the calories you eat over three or even four meals a day. You know, if you don't burneth, to fat it turneth. Now, let's continue by discussing some of the foods that are good sources of protein.

Beef and pork

"Traditionally, meat has been a popular source of protein in our diets. In recent years, a great deal of concern has been raised regarding the dangers of eating red meat. On the one hand, beef products can contain a lot of animal fat, which can raise your blood fat and cholesterol levels. This is particularly true when you eat a greasy hamburger at some burger joint where only the Great Spirit knows what's in it. On the other hand, lean red meat—and I emphasize the word lean—is less than ten percent fat and very high in protein. Lean cuts of top sirloin, flank, shank, top round, or chuck are relatively low in fat and contain about the same amount of cholesterol as skinned chicken breast. It can be an excellent source of protein. Lean cuts of venison and buffalo meat are also a good source of protein and are low in saturated fat and high in essential fatty acids. Lean pork— and I don't mean spare ribs, I mean lean pork—is abundant in protein and is lower in fat than most cuts of beef. Also, veal is lower in fat than red meat—if it isn't breaded and fried or smothered in creamy cheese or buttery sauces.

Poultry

"The white meat in chicken and turkey breast is low in fat and cholesterol and is one of the best choices of complete or whole food protein. However, the skin of these birds is high in fat and cholesterol. It's important that the skin is removed and you avoid deep fried preparations that add fat. Ground turkey and chicken burgers can be good if they're made of breast meat. However, they often contain dark meat, skin, and sometimes what only the Great Spirit knows. So be sure you're aware of the integrity of the places where you choose to eat these things.

Fish

"Fish may win the grand prize as possibly the best source of animal protein. Salmon, tuna, swordfish, halibut, and most other cold water fish are not only high in protein but also contain large amounts of essential fatty acids. They can actually encourage fat burning. Eating fish three times a week will probably provide you with all the necessary amounts of essential fatty acids you need. Fish also contain special oils that appear to prevent cardio-vascular disease. It is important to avoid adding saturated fat to your fish with deep fried preparations or sauces that smother the fish with buttery dressings. I'm often amazed at how fish can go from being a healthful food to an artery-clogging sea monster because of how it is prepared. On the other hand, baked, grilled, or pan blackened preparations with salsa or some other no fat or low-fat preparation can be absolutely delicious."

"What about shellfish, Dr. Zinney?" a thin Asian woman in her early forties asked. "My family and I really enjoy shellfish."

"Shellfish contain a substance called sterols. At one time, they were thought to cause high cholesterol; and while some authorities believe this to be exaggerated, others claim you can get 100 plus milligrams of cholesterol in a single serving of shellfish. Shellfish, like lobster and crab, are high in protein. If you eat them, avoid the fried preparations and creamy butter sauces or you will be adding a lot of saturated fat to your diet.

Non-meat protein foods

"Non-meat products, such as low-fat cottage cheese and egg whites or some commercially-prepared products made of egg whites, are chuck full of protein. Egg whites are not only a good source of protein, they're low in calories and make excellent omelets with onions, spinach, mushrooms, and salsa. Many highly competitive athletes eat no meat at all. They get all of their proteins from low-fat dairy products, eggs whites, and vegetables.

"As a side issue, consider the economics of feeding the world's population. We must feed many, many pounds of grain to cattle to produce just one pound of meat. Cattle walk, run, grow, and burn calories. You have to feed about twenty calories of grain to cattle to produce one calorie of beef. Aside from health issues, there are many people who contend that raising beef to please our palates is an uneconomical use of the resources on our planet. Lentils, soybean products, chickpeas, lima beans, navy beans, black-eyed peas, and other beans are filled with nutritious proteins. Some recent studies suggest that eating beans three times a week may decrease your chances of having a heart attack by as much as nineteen percent. Now, I don't mean refried beans—they're usually loaded with cholesterol and saturated fat."

"But, Doc, isn't it hard to get enough protein without eating meat? I mean how much protein is in beans? How much do you have to eat?" asked Craig.

"There's almost fifteen grams of protein in a cup of beans," Zinney replied. "I'm not suggesting that you have to be a vegetarian to be healthy;

but there's no doubt that you can satisfy all of your protein requirements without meat if you choose to do so."

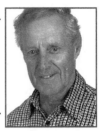

"Won't eating all those beans give us a lot of gas? I mean, I get gas from beans."

"Many vegetables, particularly beans, produce intestinal gas. To a great extent, this decreases after a few weeks of eating these foods. Your intestinal tract becomes more adept at handling them. Also, there is a product on the market called Beano that you can sprinkle on the beans that tends to reduce the gas formation. But people who have a lot of allergies, like allergy to penicillin, can have an allergy to Beano. There are also silicon products on the market that your pharmacist can recommend to decrease gaseous distention by de-foaming the gas— you know, break up the bubbles. This can allow the gas to diffuse better throughout your intestinal tract so that you have less distention. Also, tablets containing charcoal can be useful because charcoal is a potent absorbent of gas. Ask your doctor. I'm sure he or she will have good recommendations for gas.

"For you cooks, special ways of cooking the beans can also reduce gas formation. Soak the dried beans for eight hours and then slow cook them, adding a little baking soda, tomatoes, and citric acid. This seems to reduce the gas produced by beans."

Lactose intolerance

"Dr. Zinney, I don't get gas from beans, but I do seem to get a lot of gaseous distention whenever I drink milk or eat too much ice cream. What could be causing that?" asked Bertha.

"The most likely cause of gaseous distention following the ingestion of

milk products is lactose intolerance," said Zinney. "There is an enzyme in the upper part of our intestines called *lactase*. This enzyme is responsible for digesting lactose, which is the sugar present in milk products. When there is a deficiency in this enzyme, lactose is not properly digested. It undergoes fermentation resulting in excessive gaseous distention. Colicky infants occasionally have this problem for which they are given milk substitutes. They usually outgrow it by developing sufficient intestinal lactase so that they are able to drink milk and eat milk products.

"While lactose intolerance can be associated with inflammatory diseases of the bowel, it is usually a benign disturbance that is extremely common in otherwise healthy adults. There are several diagnostic tests to prove the

diagnosis of lactose intolerance; but in my experience, the simplest test is to temporarily stop using milk, ice cream, cheese, etc., and see if the gaseous symptoms disappear. Most often, the condition is easily managed by limiting the ingestion of milk products or by using milk from which the lactose has been removed.

"Fortunately, lactose free milk, or milk with reduced lactose, is available in most grocery stores. You can also purchase lactase supplements. These tablets can be taken prior to ingesting

lactose-rich products and seem to significantly reduce gaseousness in many people.

Carbohydrates

"Our discussion about the milk sugar, lactose, leads us to our next subject, carbohydrates," Zinney continued. "The beans we've just discussed, along with other vegetables and fruits, are an excellent source of carbohydrates and contain important vitamins, antioxidants, and fiber. While an important source of energy, simple sugars and refined starches, like white rice and mashed potatoes, are carbohydrates that become blood glucose. When you eat them, you have to burn them or they will turn to fat. Because carbohydrates are such an important source of energy, I recommend that about 40 percent to 60 percent of your total daily calories consist of carbohydrates. You can get this from sugar and starches like bread; but your emphasis should be on complex carbohydrates such as beans, fruits, and green vegetables. These foods contain soluble fiber that can help provide health to your intestinal tract. We'll discuss that in greater detail later."

"How about fructose? Isn't that better for you than sugar?" asked Thelma.

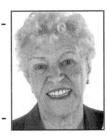

"Fructose-shmuctose—it's still sugar. Fructose, also known as levulose, is the sugar in fruits. It's a great source of energy; but please understand that if you don't burn it, it turns to fat. Burn or Blubber. Eating fruit is good because it furnishes your body with vitamins, fiber, and antioxidants; but don't delude yourself with the popularized myth that fructose has a magical quality—it's sugar. If you gorge yourself on fruit, you can get fat. You want to try to follow the food pyramid we discussed earlier. Get enough fruit in your diet; but try to make the major source of carbohydrates in your diet come from vegetables that are also high in complex carbohydrates and fiber and lower in sugar."

"Dr. Zinney, how about brown sugar and honey?" asked Thelma. "I heard they're better for you."

"Sugar is sugar is sugar. The sugar in brown sugar is sucrose, the same as in white sugar. Sucrose is cane sugar. As for honey, plants and flowers produce a thick viscous substance containing sucrose, the sugar that's in white or brown sugar. That's what the bees harvest. They convert this to fructose and glucose (also called dextrose)—that's honey. Athletes believe it to be a good source of energy because glucose provides immediate energy and fructose can be readily stored as glycogen providing a more delayed source of energy. But you have to get rid of the myth—it's still sugar. You either burn it and pump up or you don't and you blubber up. To some extent, sugar is okay; but again, it's best to get most of your carbohydrates in the form of complex carbs that are high in fiber.

Fats

"Let's talk a little about fat. All of you remember that there are nine calories in every gram of fat—more than twice the number of calories as in proteins and carbohydrates. That's not all the bad news. Fat can clog up your arteries resulting in heart attacks and strokes. But not all kinds of fat are bad. Your body needs certain essential fatty acids for health; and as we said earlier, we can get lots of those from fish. The major culprits are the fats found in meat and dairy products, the saturated fats. Most of the fats found in vegetables are unsaturated fats. They are the polyunsaturated fats and mono-unsaturated fats, like in gua-camole and macadamia nuts. They're the good guys. But they're still fats and they still have all those calories.

"It's also important to note that there are some fats from the vegetable world that are dangerous and you should avoid them, such as coconut oil and palm oil. Some artificial creamers use these. Some vegetable fats may actual-ly help lower your blood triglycerides and cholesterol and protect you against heart disease. Olive oil, sesame oil, canola oil, and safflower oil are examples of good guys. But please, please don't forget that they have nine calories per gram, more than twice the amount that proteins and carbohy-drates have."

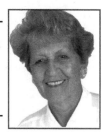

"Dr. Zinney, how much fat or cholesterol can we be allowed in our diet?" Miriam asked.

"I was just going to get to that," Zinney responded. "On a daily basis, I don't think you should have more than 30 percent of your calories come from fat. Moreover, you should try to keep your saturated fat intake lower than 10 percent of your daily calories. Many studies suggest that younger people are at much greater risk from elevated blood cholesterol levels than older people. Elevated cholesterol is a major risk factor for the development of coronary artery disease and heart attacks, particularly in middle-aged men and women.

"In older ages, elevated cholesterol lev-els appear to be a minor risk factor. Because of this, some have concluded that older people don't have to restrict their cholesterol. I don't agree. There is no good reason to continue a bad habit because someone else has decid-ed that the damage is already done and says that it won't affect your longevity. As an individual, it can affect your longevity and your vitality. You're going to live longer than the preceding generation; and the genera-tion following you will live longer than your generation. The so-called middle age period of life will be rede-fined. Many of the terrible effects that high cholesterol has on our blood ves-sels can be stayed and even reversed by a low cholesterol intake and exercise. Don't give up on yourself. Limit your cholesterol intake to 100 mil-ligrams a day."

"Doc, Kinder here again. I hear people talking about cholesterol, triglycerides, and fiber all the time. I think I know what fiber is but I'm not quite sure. And I don't get this stuff I hear about good and bad cholesterol or why it's important. What is all this stuff?"

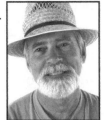

Cholesterol

"Cholesterol is important fat-like stuff manufactured by your liver and also present in many foods. So the cholesterol in your blood is derived from two basic sources: the cholesterol you eat and the cholesterol your liver manufactures. In some people, their liver makes very little cholesterol and they can gorge themselves on food that is high in cholesterol and still have normal blood levels. All of us know someone who can eat bacon and eggs and steak, ice cream, and chocolates in large amounts every day and never have a cholesterol problem. We envy them! Other people can severely restrict their cholesterol intake; but, because their liver makes so much cholesterol, they still have elevated blood cholesterol. It's possible that your genes determine and control the amount of cholesterol your liver makes."

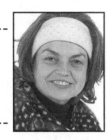

"Why do we have cholesterol? What does it do?" asked Sheila.

"The fat-like substance we call cholesterol is important. It is used by our bodies to help manufacture hormones and the membranes of our cells. When the blood level gets too high, above two hundred, it can accumulate on the walls of our arteries and cause heart attacks and strokes.

"Egg yolk and dairy products are examples of high cholesterol foods. Red meat, the skin on chicken and turkey, and the dark meat of these birds contain more cholesterol than you need. Organs like liver, brain, pancreas, and thymus gland are also high in cholesterol and possibly some shellfish as well. So a low cholesterol diet is low in dairy products, red meat, and egg yolks and high in fish, the white meat of chicken and turkey, and fruits and vegetables."

Good cholesterol and bad cholesterol

"Ok, Doc," said Kinder, "but what is this stuff about good and bad cholesterol and triglycerides?"

89

"It's important that you know there is no good cholesterol in the food you eat. There's no food source for good cholesterol, also known as HDL. In other words, you can't eat good cholesterol; you have to make it.

"Let me explain. Special carriers in our blood stream transport cholesterol throughout our body. They're called lipoproteins, the most important of which are called low-density lipoproteins or LDL (bad cholesterol), very low-density lipoproteins or VLDL , and high-density lipoproteins or HDL (good cholesterol). For the most part, the LDL is the bad cholesterol that clogs up the arteries and causes heart attacks and strokes by closing the artery off. Eating too much cholesterol is the major cause of this. But as discussed earlier, in some people genetics play a very important role.

"Good cholesterol, or HDL, may actually remove bad cholesterol from the walls of the arteries and bring it to the liver where it may be metabolized or harmlessly excreted into the bile. Exercising, losing weight, and quitting smoking can all have a dramatic effect on increasing the levels of good cholesterol. For good health, we like to see the total cholesterol below 200 and the bad cholesterol or LDL below 130 and the good cholesterol above 30 or 35. Most of you can achieve this with diet and exercise. In those cases where diet and exercise does not produce the desired effect, your doctor can prescribe cholesterol-lowering medications that have proven to be very effective.

C-Reactive protein (CRP)

"Many authorities believe that inflammation plays an important role in the development of heart attacks. To check this belief, they measured markers in the blood for inflammation and found them to be elevated in many who went on to have a heart attack, even in the presence of normal levels of bad cholesterol. These markers, in the absence of other causes for inflammation such as infection or recent trauma, appear to be quite accurate predictors of cardiac risk. One of the best tests, or markers, is the determination of C-reactive protein. This test is readily available and easily performed. You might ask your doctor about adding it to your cardiac risk assessment."

Triglycerides

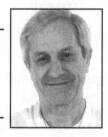

"Doc, you mentioned triglycerides earlier. I'd like you to tell us about them."

"Be happy to," Zinney responded. "The significance of triglycerides—

90

the other fat substance circulating in our blood, is somewhat controversial. High levels do appear to be a risk factor for heart attacks, particularly among women. And more recently, high triglyceride levels have been linked to an increase in the frequency of strokes. Triglyceride levels often decrease when the good cholesterol (HDL) levels increase. So you see, Sam, a good diet and exercise can also be effective in decreasing your triglyceride levels. I can see by your head nodding that you get it.

Zinney's zummary

"So in conclusion, you should get about 40 to 50 percent of your calories from carbohydrates—mostly high fiber carbs and 20 to 30 percent from proteins and no more than 30 percent from fats. Try to keep the animal fat low, at less than ten percent. As Dr. Christian Barnard said, 'die young as late as possible.' Eating the correct heart-friendly foods can go a long way in making this happen. Eat a diet that is rich in fruits and vegetables. They contain fiber, vitamins, minerals, and the antioxidants as well as other healthful things. For example, purple grape juice and red wine are loaded with chemicals called flavinoids. They can thin the blood and improve the elasticity of blood vessels. Oranges, apricots, and bananas are rich in

potassium, which can help lower blood pressure. Less common fruits like pomegranates contain an enzyme called paroxonase that can break up plaques on our arteries.

"Try to limit your intake of the saturated fat contained in most red meat and dairy products. Use poultry and fish as your main source of protein. If you're a committed carnivore, and you have to eat red meat, try grass-fed beef or even wild game like venison instead of the traditional grain-fed beef. The corrrect foods are higher in the polyunsaturated omega three oils. These oils improve the flexibility of arteries and may even reduce the inflammatory reaction of blood vessels. You can find lots of them in fish, canola oil, walnuts, and flaxseed.

"The worst are the hydrogenated vegetable oils. They are made of the *transfats*. These not only raise your level of LDL, the bad cholesterol; but they can also decrease your level of HDL, the good cholesterol. So limit your intake of these oils. Try to substitute them with the mono-unsaturated fats in things like avocados and olive oil and the polyunsaturated fats. I said earlier that there are no food sources that can give you HDL, the good cholesterol. However, some heart-friendly foods have the tendency to both decrease your bad cholesterol and

91

increase your good cholesterol. Olive oil and the organo-sulfurs in onions might do this. And please, read the labels on the foods you buy. Try to stay away from too many chemicals or preservatives.

"Once again, my friends, we've run out of time. Next week we'll answer the other part of John's question, the part about dietary fiber. I also want to tell you about the importance of vitamin and mineral supplements and discuss any other kind of supplements you might be interested in knowing about. Have a healthy week and give some thought to your dietary supplements. How much fiber do we need? What vitamins or herbs should we be taking or not taking? These are good questions with very important answers. Good night, and thank you again for being here."

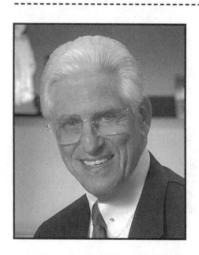

7

Now the saga shall begin
About your favorite vitamin.
Is what you know about your herb
A "not so scientific" blurb?

Fiber, Vitamins, and Herbs

Ms. Worthington remained seated in the front row as the auditorium filled. Observing that the audience consisted of mostly familiar faces, she felt comfortable having Dr. Zinney introduce himself. "Good evening," Zinney began. "It's nice to see you folks again. I also see a few newcomers here tonight. I'm Dr. Zinney, and I'm glad you could join us."

"Tonight I'm going to tell you what you need to know about fiber and fluids. We're also going to talk about vitamins, minerals and herbs. So, all of you listen in; and if you have any questions, just raise your hand and I'll try to find you.

The scoop on poop

"Since what we put in our mouths has a monumental effect on what comes out of our backside, particularly in the case of fiber, I feel compelled to start this discussion bass-ackwards. So, let's talk a little about *caca* with a brief review of stool formation and evacuation. I am puzzled as to why Nature had made this exciting and physiologically beautiful act have, as its end-product, that which can be so malodorous and uncomely in appearance, but so be it.

"Ingested food is propelled through the digestive tract by contractions of the muscles within its walls. These delicately coordinated muscular contractions are called peristalsis. Digestion of the food we eat and absorption of nutrients from that food takes place as the food passes through our stomachs and our small intestines. The residual material, feces, is passed into the colon; as it advances, water is absorbed, causing the stool to solidify. The feces are then moved further along into the rectum by contractions of the colon (peristalsis). When the amount of feces in the lower colon and rectum reaches a critical point, the urge to defecate becomes apparent.

"The voluntary act of defecation is comprised of several components. It begins with a forceful bearing down together with contraction of the diaphragm and the abdominal musculature. This causes an increase in intra-abdominal pressure. The increasing intra-abdominal pressure together with increased peristalsis gets things ready to blow. This is followed, almost immediately, by an exquisitely coordinated reflex in the ano-rectal area consisting of relaxation of the anal sphincters and elevation of the anus by a muscle called the *levator ani*. Under normal circumstances, the events that follow might be best described as a series of ka-plunkety plops, as the stool then drops.

Acute constipation

"Let me say a few words about acute constipation before discussing the chronic form that plagues so many people. A change in bowel habit or any new recurrent change can signal the presence of a mechanical obstruction to the flow of stool. This might be caused by a tumor or inflammatory narrowing. Sudden or recurrent changes, whether in the form of constipation or diarrhea, should be evaluated by a physician without undue delay.

Chronic constipation

"That said, we know that if you don't get enough fiber and water in your diet you're likely to suffer from constipation. Moreover, it's likely to worsen as you age. This may take the form of difficulty in passing stool, infrequent bowel movements (fewer than three a week), or a feeling of incomplete evacuation. The frequent straining at stool may result in hemorrhoids, painful fissures or cracks around the anus, the development of diverticulosis, or the extrusion of some of the lining of the rectum, a condition called rectal prolapse.

"Weakness of any of the musculature involved in the act of defecation or any disease process that affects the neuromuscular activity of these muscles or the intrinsic muscles of the colon, can be responsible for chronic constipation. As an example, weakness of the abdominal muscles or weakness of the muscles of the pelvic floor may contribute to constipation. Many authorities believe that a very distressing, but relatively benign, condition called the Irritable Bowel Syndrome is the result of a defect in the neuromuscular activity of the intestinal wall. This condition can cause constipation, diarrhea, or both.

"In addition, any of the following factors can cause constipation: lack of exercise, a diet low in fiber, inadequate fluid intake, laxative abuse, the use of constipating medications, and the habitual postponement of the urge to defecate. Recognizing that such a large variety of issues can contribute to constipation underscores the need for people with this condition to have a thorough physical examination. While your physician may be reassuring, he or she may recommend additional tests such as sigmoidoscopy, colonoscopy, x-rays, or other special tests depending on the individual circumstances of your case."

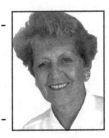

"You mentioned constipating medications. What kind do you mean?" asked Miriam.

"The list of medications that can cause or contribute to constipation is a mile long," said Zinney. "It can range from antacids you might take for dyspepsia to the side effects of any medications that alter bowel activity. Narcotics and other pain relievers, bowel-relaxing drugs called anticholinergics and even some tranquilizers are examples. It's a good reason to check with your doctor if you develop constipation while taking medications.

"Fortunately, we have the ability to deny the urge to go to stool because the external anal sphincter is under our voluntary control. However, the frequent and habitual denial of the urge to use the toilet can cause chronic constipation. Prolonged retention of the stool allows more water to be absorbed and the stool becomes harder. More stool may enter the area and more denial causes more hardening. When you finally go to the toilet, you grunt and groan and strain. If this becomes routine, the rectum acclimates to an increased volume of hard stool and is less and less sensitive to the presence of stool. The normal signal to evacuate can become delayed and a vicious cycle that ends in the development of chronic constipation is the result.

"Should this be taken to the extreme, the compacted stool can become voluminous, causing what is referred to as fecal impaction. Fecal impactions can fill and obstruct the rectum. This can necessitate a visit to the emergency room where an oil retention enema, followed by a digital disimpaction, is performed to remove the stool from the rectum—not a pleasant experience. Fecal impactions are particularly common among the elderly as a result of dehydration coupled with a sluggish bowel. It may also frequent hospitalized patients because of the inactivity imposed by bed rest, the use of medications which may be constipating, and the fact that they find themselves in an unfamiliar environment. Unfamiliarity with one's surroundings can cause a conscious or unconscious delay in using the toilet. So you see, my friends, promptly responding to the urge to defecate, adequate fluid intake, and avoiding inactivity through regular exercise are important tools in the prevention of constipation.

Laxatives and enemas

"Many people seek to alleviate their constipation by taking laxatives or enemas. While the occasional use of laxatives or enemas to solve the occasional problem is sometimes useful, the more you take, the more you need. The neuromuscular complexes that are responsible for normal defecation can become dependent on the stimulation produced by the frequent use of laxatives and enemas.

"You want to avoid getting into a situation where defecation reflexes require laxative stimulation. If you're already there, you may need to retrain your colon by gradually tapering off laxative use and increasing your intake of fiber and fluids."

"How about high colonic cleansing enemas?" asked Bertha. "They're supposed to clean out the toxins."

"The only thing they clean out is your wallet," Zinney responded. "There are no toxins and, besides that, the colon cleanses itself by regenerating most of its lining every twenty-four hours. The value of a high colonic cleansing enema is a myth without any scientific merit. It's a fairy tale perpetuated on an unknowing public—but now you're informed, so don't use them."

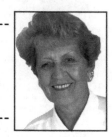

"Are there any laxatives that are more safe to take than others?" asked Miriam.

"That's a good question, Miriam," responded Zinney. "If you must use laxatives, use the mildest one that works for you and use it for the shortest period of time possible. That having been said, laxatives can be classified into different categories depending on their mechanism of action.

There are hyperosmolar and saline laxatives, irritant laxatives, bulk forming laxatives, and stool softeners.

"*Irritant laxatives* such as Dulcolax, Senokot, Ex-lax, and Feen-a-mint actually irritate the lining of the colon and stimulate expulsive contractions. These are often associated with cramping, abdominal discomfort, loss of nutrients, and a proclivity to produce dependence.

"*Hyperosmolar laxatives* consist of mixed electrolyte solutions containing polyethelene glycol or nonabsorbable sugars like lactulose or sorbitol. They cause an outpouring of fluid into the colon increasing the pressure inside the colon and liquifying the stool. They are used primarily for cleansing the bowel for diagnostic procedures. However, Miralax, which contains polyethelene glycol, or lactulose, a nonabsorbable sugar, is occasionally prescribed in severe chronic constipation.

"*Saline laxatives* are very popular. The most commonly used is Milk of Magnesia. Like the hyperosmolar laxatives discussed, they also work by pulling fluid into your colon. This makes the stool softer and easier to pass. The frequent use of saline cathartics can cause fluid retention in the elderly, a serious problem for people with high blood pressure, kidney, or cardiovascular disorders. They should not be used on a regular basis.

"*Stool softeners* are not really purgatives. They don't actually cause you to have a bowel movement. They soften the stool making it easier to pass. Stool softeners are not harmful, but they can cause you to stain your undergarments because of occasional inadvertent passage of stool. Some popular examples are Colace, Dialose, and Surfak. Mineral oil is both a laxative and a stool softener. It can lubricate the bowel and soften the stool, but it can also interfere with the absorption of nutrients, particularly the fat-soluable vitamins. Rarely, people who have difficulty swallowing may aspirate some into their lungs resulting in a nasty condition called lipid pneumonia. For these reasons, it's best used as a retention enema to soften hard stools. When taken orally, it should be used sparingly and only taken on an empty stomach at bedtime.

"*Bulkforming laxatives*, because they consist of some form of plant fiber, are safer than most others. Popular brands such as Metamucil, Serutan, and Citrucel probably account for 15 to 30 percent of laxative use in the U.S.A. They facilitate the passage of stool by drawing water into the colon and absorbing that water. This makes the stool softer and larger and easier to pass. However, it's essential to take a full glass of water with bulk formers to avoid hardening of the stool. It's also important that they be used an hour or two after any other medications to avoid interfering with the absorption of the medicine."

Fiber

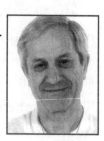

"Well, you told us about how to crap and how not to crap," said Sam. "But we still don't know very much about fiber or how much water we should be drinking."

"Okay, Sam. Let's begin with fiber. The fiber in plants, like vegetables and fruits, is the stuff that gives the plant its strength and its structure. It's like the skeleton of the plant. It's the part of the vegetable or fruit that can't be digested.

"Most fruits and vegetables contain soluble fiber and insoluble fiber. They both benefit us in somewhat different ways. The difference between them is really simple. *Soluble fiber* is fiber that can dissolve in water and *insoluble fiber* is fiber that will not dissolve in water. Let's take a look at the diagram of the intestinal tract in this next slide [fig. 7A].

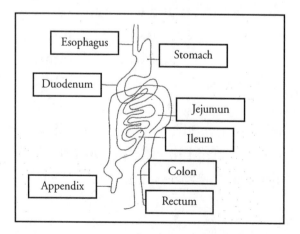

"Insoluble fiber adds bulk to the stool in the lower intestine by absorbing water and in this way speeds up the progress of waste material through the colon. Soluble fiber slows the emptying of the stomach and the motility of the small bowel producing an increased sense of satiety or fullness— a greater sense of satisfaction. Because of its gelling properties, it also aids in the regulation of glucose absorption.

"Bulk formation is further increased because of the ability of soluble fiber to absorb water and encourage bacterial fermentation. These actions improve the lubrication of waste; they improve the transit time in the colon by enhancing motor activity or peristalsis; and they decrease the pressure within the colon."

"Dr. Zinney!" Bertha interrupted. "What does this fermentation you're talking about mean? And, how does that help us?"

"Bacteria are normally present inside the colon or large intestine. The action of the bacteria on soluble fiber is known as fermentation. In addition to increasing bulking, fermentation of carbohydrates and amino acids results in *fatty acids*. Fatty acids are an energy source for colon cells and may prevent colon cancer. They also appear to

Fig 7A

improve the liver's ability to metabolize fats and glucose."

"Dr. Zinney," said John Kinder, "I don't understand all that stuff about decreasing pressure in the colon and fermentation and those fatty acid things. And what's more important, I still don't understand how fiber helps us."

"Well, John, it can be a little complicated and maybe it needs more explanation," replied Zinney. "Let me take another and more simple crack at it. Both soluble and insoluble fiber are important, but soluble fiber seems to play a greater role in the prevention and treatment of many diseases. In addition to absorbing water and producing bulk, soluble fiber enters into a chemical reaction with the bacteria in the colon. This chemical reaction is a fermentation process like the kind that curdles milk or the kind that is used to make wine. The fermentation reaction in the colon produces stuff called fatty acids that may protect the colon from cancer and may also improve the metabolism of glucose and fat by the liver. Additionally, the bulk formed by the absorption of water by the fiber improves the transportation of waste and decreases the pressure in the colon and rectum."

Fiber content of food

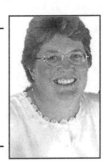

"How much fiber are we supposed to eat and what foods contain the right kind of fiber?" inquired Bertha.

"Bertha, a lot of folks are confused about the fiber content in different foods. As an example, many harbor the misconception that there's a lot of fiber in lettuce when, in fact, there's very little fiber value in lettuce. That said, most high fiber foods contain both soluble and insoluble fiber. Nuts, dried beans, whole grain cereals, wheat bran and many other vegetables are good sources. Oat bran and psyllium are particularly good sources of soluble fiber. [See page 115 for a chart showing the fiber content of selected foods.]

"People are also confused in regard to the amount of fiber they should be eating. The average American diet contains about 10-15 grams of fiber a day but we really should be eating as much as 25-30 grams a day."

"Jeez!" commented Sam. "If I ate 30 grams of fiber, I'd get rabbit ears and grow tulips out my backside."

Fluids

"Honey, you already have rabbit ears and you already have huge purple tulips growing out your backside.

They're hemorrhoids from not eating enough fiber and not drinking enough water. You know the doctor told you to drink six to eight glasses of water a day," replied Sheila.

"Not really," said Sam. "He said to drink six glasses of *fluid* a day."

"I was right there," she retorted. "He said six to eight glasses of non-alcoholic and non-caffeinated beverages. To me, that means water or juices—not booze or coffee. He said people should drink that much unless they have a water retention problem like from kidney, heart, or liver disease. Then, they should check with their doctor to determine how much they should drink."

"C'mon, Sheila, what's wrong with coffee or booze?" asked Sam.

"Caffeine and alcohol can make you squirt out as much or more fluid as you take in," replied Sheila. "You know that, Sam. Why don't you ask Zinney. Go ahead and ask Zinney."

"Ok, I will," said Sam. "Dr. Z, how much fluid should we be drinking a day?"

"This will vary from one individual to the next. A person's size, physical activity, and climatic conditions are important determinants," Zinney answered. "The hotter and drier the climate and greater the physical activity, the greater our fluid requirement. While I too have heard that everyone should have about six to eight glasses of water a day, I don't know the scientific basis for that recommendation. Use common sense; if you're thirsty, drink some water! I should emphasize though, that with hot days and physical exertion, you should increase your fluid intake. You should be able to satisfy your fluid requirements by drinking water and other beverages and also from the food you eat."

John Kinder jumped in, "How about coffee? Does coffee count?"

"Insightful question, John! Beverages containing caffeine like coffee or even tea don't count as much. Caffeine is a diuretic and so is alcohol. They can cause the kidneys to work overtime and may even cause you to lose fluid. Fruit juices are a good source of fluids and are packed with vitamins, but you do have to watch the calories.

"While drinking water is the best way of making sure your fluid intake is adequate, there's lots of water in the food you eat, particularly in vegetables and fruits. Drinking water is good;

but drinking eight glasses of water on top of a healthful fluid-rich food intake can be a little much for some people, particularly those with heart, kidney or liver problems. These folks should check with their doctor in regard to their fluid requirements."

The benefits of fiber

"Dr. Zinney," said Craig. "Now that we know more about the fiber and fluids we need, could you tell us more about what diseases we're curing or preventing with fiber?"

"Ok, Craig. Let's start with the colon and rectum. Colon polyps are benign tumors. Some of them, however, may become or turn into colon cancer. In fact, it's believed that most colon cancers begin as benign polyps. There is a lot of scientific evidence that dietary fiber reduces the development of polyps, thus also reducing the chances of colon cancer."

"I heard that some recent studies disproved the protective effect that fiber was supposed to have on colon cancer," said Craig. "Would you comment on that, Dr. Zinney?"

"Well, they haven't exactly disproved it," said Zinney. "But it's a very good point and it warrants explanation. Some very well done studies have recently shown that a high fiber diet, taken for four years, did not prevent recurrent polyps during that four-year period. I emphasize the word recur-

rent. All of the people in the study had polyps previously.

"This suggests, that they either had a genetic proclivity to develop polyps or they might have done dietary damage to their colon or both. The studies showed that in these subjects a high fiber intake did not prevent recurrence of polyps during those four years. It doesn't mean that it wouldn't have prevented the frequency of recurrent polyps over a longer period of time—say, twenty years.

"On the flip side, many observational studies strongly suggest that a high fiber diet is protective against developing colon tumors. It has been noted that colon tumors are very uncommon in certain parts of the world, like Africa and Asia, where diets are high in fiber. It has also been observed that when people from Asia and Africa immigrate to our country and adopt our low fiber dietary habits, their frequency of colon tumors begins to increase and approximate the overall incidence seen in this country. Despite this, there is much yet to be learned on this subject. Whether you believe fiber protects against colon tumors or not, there's a multitude of other very good reasons to eat a high fiber diet. Let's discuss some now.

Hemorrhoids

"We know that fiber absorbs water, lubricates the stool, and promotes or enhances peristalsis—the propulsive motor activity of the colon. In this way, fiber decreases the pressure in the colon and rectum. As a result of decreasing the internal pressures, the development of both diverticulosis and hemorrhoids are decreased."

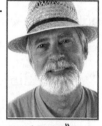

"We hear a lot about diverticulosis, but I don't really know what that is," said John. "And how does decreasing the pressure in the colon prevent it or hemorrhoids?"

"Good question again, John. We'll start with hemorrhoids. Normally we have these little anal cushions filled with tiny blood vessels in our rectum, down near the anus [fig. 7B]. As the pressure in the rectum increases, the shearing force on these anal cushions increases. Over time, this increased shearing force causes the supporting tissues around these anal cushions to weaken and develop into hemorrhoids. With continued pressure, the hemorrhoids get larger and larger and more engorged with blood. And as the supporting structures become weaker and weaker, the hemorrhoids continue to enlarge and may even prolapse or telescope downwards and even protrude out the anus. Some people have to actually push them back up with their fingers after a bowel movement.

"Sometimes the condition progresses to the extent that they get stuck and can't be pushed back and need surgery. As hemorrhoids enlarge, the lining of the rectum and anus covering the hemorrhoids gets stretched and the hemorrhoids may become painful or itch or bleed."

"That's what my doctor says is wrong with me," Craig whispered to Sam. "He says I have a very bad case of Zakley. I'll bet that's what you have."

"What the heck is Zakley?" Sam asked.

"That's when your backside looks e-Zakley like your face," laughed Craig.

"Dr. Zinney, I hear people talk about internal hemorrhoids and external hemorrhoids. What's the difference?" asked Bertha.

"The last part of the rectum, or the anal canal, is lined by tissue that is similar to skin as you can see in the slide [fig. 7B].

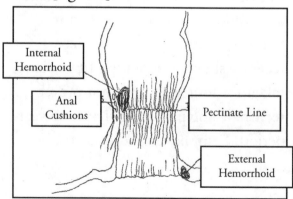

Fig 7B

"The line that divides the upper and lower parts of the rectum and anal canal is the *pectinate line*. If a hemorrhoid develops above this line, it's called an internal hemorrhoid; and if it develops below the line, it's an external hemorrhoid.

"Since an external hemorrhoid is covered by skin-like tissue, it can itch and become very painful. Sometimes, a blood clot forms inside the hemorrhoid and has to be surgically evacuated.

"So you see, Bertha, external hemorrhoids can be very painful; but because of their thick covering of skin, they don't usually bleed. They're more apt to cause pain and itching. On the other hand, internal hemorrhoids are formed above the pectinate line. They are covered by the same kind of lining as the colon. This is a thinner covering and has little or no pain nerves. So they have a greater tendency to bleed, very often without causing any pain or discomfort. A high fiber diet and a good fluid intake can decrease the internal pressure in the colon and rectum. If we decrease the pressure, we decrease the shearing force we talked about. This may prevent hemorrhoids or reduce their severity after they have developed.

Diverticulosis

"Let's get on with diverticulosis of the colon. These are small pouches or pockets that form at weak points in the colon. Most physicians believe that low fiber diets are primarily responsible for causing diverticulosis. A diet low in fiber causes the internal pressure in the colon to increase. This causes the muscles in the wall of the colon to strain and increase in thickness. Weak spots then form between these thickened bands of muscle. The increase in internal pressure in the colon then causes the weak spots in the colon to bulge outward and form pockets or diverticula [fig. 7C].

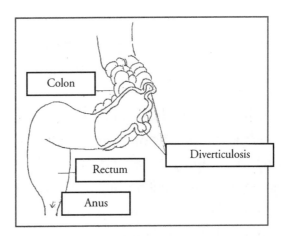

"Interestingly, diverticulosis is most prevalent in well-developed industrialized populations of the world, like the United States and England, and hardly problematic in less-developed countries. The condition became most evident at about the same time refined flour and other processed foods were introduced, in the early 1900s. Whole-wheat flour has an abundance of bran whereas refined flour has no wheat bran. In less developed areas like Africa and Asia, diverticulosis is rare. In these areas, the diet is abundant in unprocessed foods and fiber."

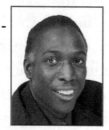

"Dr. Zinney, my name is Leonard Johnson. I think you're right. Most of my family still lives in Africa and nobody ever had this condition. But my uncle who came here almost seventy years ago was diagnosed with diverticulitis last week. What's the difference between diverticulosis, diverticula, and diverticulitis?"

"Ok, Leonard. Lots of people have trouble keeping these terms straight. One of these pockets or pouches is called a diverticulum. The term *diverticula* is the plural form and *diverticulum*, the singular. *Diverticulosis* is the name given to the condition of having diverticula. People with diverticulosis may not have any symptoms and might not even know they have the condition. However, sometimes diverticulosis is associated with bloating and constipation along with mild to moderate abdominal discomfort and cramping. When diverticula become infected and inflamed, the condition is called *diverticulitis*. It's diverticulosis when there is no inflammation or infection and diverticulitis when there is.

"Diverticulitis can be a very serious problem. Most of the time, this infection can be cleared up in a few days with antibiotics. But sometimes, an abscess forms or the infected diverticula perforate like a ruptured appendix. This allows pus to spill into the abdomen, causing peritonitis. These are very serious complications and often require surgery.

"Also bleeding can occur from diverticula, sometimes quite severe. The bleeding is believed to come from the rupture of tiny, weakened blood vessels in the diverticula. While this usually stops on its own, on rare occasions it can be life threatening; and blood transfusions or surgery may be necessary. So you see folks, it would be good to follow a high fiber diet and prevent the development of diverticulosis. For those of us who already have diverticulosis, a high fiber diet may decrease the likelihood of these miserable complications."

Fiber and diabetes

"Dr. Zinney, Leonard again. My son is in medical school and he talks about this stuff all the time, but I usually don't understand most of what he's talking about. I'm a diabetic and he's always telling me that increasing my fiber can help me lose weight and help control my diabetes. Is this true?"

"Leonard, it sounds like your son is going to be a good doctor. Since soluble fiber slows the emptying of your stomach, it can help produce a sense of satiety or satisfaction. This can assist you in taking in less food, making it easier to lose weight and to follow your diabetic diet. Also, as we discussed earlier, soluble fiber has a gelling action, which can smooth out the absorption of carbs and sugars. This decreases the roller coaster effect of high sugar—high insulin and fat formation. But you see, soluble fiber benefits more than just your diabetes and your blood sugar.

"Soluble fiber can also reduce the absorption of fat and cholesterol so it can help lower your cholesterol and reduce your risk of a heart attack. In this regard, Leonard, your son has given you good advice. Let me give you some more advice: follow your son's advice. All of us should take about 25 grams to 30 grams of fiber a day. If you don't get enough of it in your food, like in vegetables, fruits, nuts, or oat bran, ask your doctor for help. He or she might recommend psyllium or some other fiber supplement. Speaking of supplements, let's talk about them for a bit.

Herbs and mega dose vitamins

"For several years, physicians were taught that a nutritious diet obviated the need for dietary supplements. We were taught that there were enough vitamins and minerals in a healthful diet so that taking extra vitamins had the effect of producing expensive urine but did not add to the health of the individual. In other words, the body would take and use what it needed, and the rest would be excreted in the urine or not even absorbed and passed in the stool. In days gone by, conventional wisdom sometimes even condemned the use of supplemental vitamins except in cases of vitamin deficiencies. Such deficiencies could result from inborn errors in absorption, metabolism, or disease states that could cause wasting or poor absorption of nutrients.

"To a large extent, the pendulum has swung in an equally inappropriate direction and should be brought more closely back to the midline. It is now commonplace for people to gulp a handful of vitamins and herbs on a daily basis harboring the sincere belief that these pills and powders will improve their memory, strength, potency, and longevity. This is the result of good marketing. People who market these supplements have convinced some of us that we need these expensive supplements to restore strength and youthful energy.

"The fact is, the ingredients in many of the items touted at some health food stores can be purchased at a drugstore for a fraction of the price. Moreover, the safety and the value of many of these supplements may not have been scientifically established. They don't fall under the province of FDA evaluation, and false claims based on less-than-good scientific study are often made. These claims may enormously exaggerate the importance of the stuff some sales clerks are hawking. Many supplements sold by scientific-sounding clerks at health food stores may actually be harmful. Others that would normally be harmless may interfere with the action of certain medications. So check with your doctor before taking any of these herbs or supplements and don't part with your money too quickly."

"Ok, Dr. Zinney, but what about vitamins and the other antioxidants?" asked Miriam. "I heard that vitamin C helps to prevent colds and also that antioxidants help to prevent aging and vitamin D helps to prevent fractures. Is all this bunk or what? You hear it from everybody."

"You're right, Miriam. You do hear it everywhere and there is some truth to some of it. Conventional wisdom is changing in favor of taking certain supplements as a result of increasing scientific information, but definitely NOT to the extent of taking mega doses of vitamins or a handful of herbs each day. Even the best of intentions from the non-medical community should be viewed with skepticism.

Too much vitamin C

"Take vitamin C as an example. A brilliant non-physician Nobel laureate thought that vitamin C would prevent colds and he recommended that we take 500 milligrams or more a day. Some people were taking 1000 milligrams and even 2000 milligrams a day. It had become a very popular thing to do. Now, a recent scientific study suggested that taking more than 500 milligrams of vitamin C each day might cause thickening of your coronary arteries. Larger doses may cause diarrhea and kidney stones. Moreover, numerous scientifically performed studies have dispelled the myth that vitamin C prevents colds. You've got to realize you can get too much of a good thing. Vitamin C is good for you but don't take more than 500 milligrams a day.

Too much vitamin A

"Vitamin A is another example. Because vitamin A tends to accumulate in the liver and because it is so easily absorbed, the elderly are particularly vulnerable to vitamin A toxicity. Acute overloading can cause diarrhea, nausea, dizziness, drowsiness and later enlargement of the liver and spleen. As an example, a severe and almost fatal illness reportedly developed among a group of explorers from eating polar bear liver, which has a very high concentration of vitamin A.

"That said, even mild overdosing over a long period of time can be hazardous. Recent studies have demonstrated a high incidence of bone fractures in folks taking more than 2800 International Units a day. It appears that if we take too much as a long-term daily supplement, vitamin A can make our bones fragile. This calls into question the purpose of having high concentrations in our multivitamin pills and the wisdom of our fortifying so many foods with vitamin A. Vitamin A is an important antioxidant and it's good for you. Among other things, it can help prevent night blindness and deterioration of the cornea; but read those labels and try not to take more than 2800 IU a day. As an aside, I might add that an International Unit is simply a unit of measurement that tells us the quantity and potency of a vitamin.

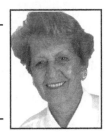

"So all this herb and vitamin stuff is a bunch of hogwash?" asked Miriam.

"That's not what I mean, Miriam. Don't get me wrong. I'm not against taking vitamins or herbs or certain supplements. I am against taking too much of the right thing and any of the wrong thing. You should get most of your vitamins from a balanced diet and supplement vitamins and minerals based on scientific evidence. Now, there are some of us who are on some crazy fad diet to lose weight. Then there are the many others of us who just don't eat enough fresh vegetables, fruits, and fish. Taking a small multivitamin supplement, calcium with vitamin D, one natural vitamin E pill of 400 IU and 250mg of vitamin C is generally considered to be a safe way to solve most of the problems that might be associated with a less than healthful diet.

Herbs

"The study of herbs has given rise to many important discoveries and doubtless there will be many more in the future. Heart medications like digitalis and pain relievers derived from opium are obvious examples. Herbal remedies have been used for centuries and undoubtedly some of these herbs are effective—but many are not.

"It's now popular to take herbs to improve your memory, the health of your prostate, your sexuality, and your immune system. Lots of luck.

"Discuss your need for any of these things with your doctor. The important thing is to produce maximum benefit with a minimum risk of doing harm.

"While it's true that it often takes ten years for a scientific discovery or theory to get to the point of public consumption, please be careful. While many herbs may be of benefit, many others are not, despite so-called scientific claims to the contrary. Often these scientific claims are not so scientific. If the benefits of taking something are not clearly and scientifically demonstrated and the risks of taking it have not been thoroughly evaluated, then *please* don't take it.

"Even worse, some dietary supplements and so-called herbs actually contain raw animal parts. A bottle labeled 'thymus' may contain bovine lymphoid tissue rather than the herb thyme. The term *orchis* can be easily mistaken for a plant herb instead of an extract from the testicle of a bull.

In one case, extracts from seventeen different bovine organs, with ingredients from spleen, brain, lymph glands, and pituitary glands were found in a supplement. What about people who have religious restrictions against eating these things? What about vegetarians who would find eating dead cow parts disgusting? Shouldn't the list of ingredients be complete? Still more disconcerting, these ingredients may be imported from foreign countries and susceptible to all kinds of contamination, including the agents that cause mad cow disease.

"Presently, the Department of Agriculture's surveillance on imported substances applies only to those that are used in food and medicines and not to those that are used in dietary supplements. This is a catastrophe waiting to happen. Again, if the risks or benefits of taking something are not firmly and scientifically established, then please don't take it.

"Remember, eating a healthful diet and, with some exceptions, taking the supplements described, will provide you with a substantial and safe vitamin and mineral intake. Now let's get more specific and begin by discussing some of the important B vitamins.

Vitamin B12, folic acid, and vitamin B6

"With advancing age, the lining of the gastrointestinal tract can get thin; it begins to wear out. When this occurs in the stomach, the condition is called atrophic gastritis; and this condition is often associated with a decrease in the absorption of B12 and also of folic acid. Leafy vegetables, fruits, and yeast are good sources of folic acid or folate. But if your ability to absorb folate decreases, you might not get enough of this B vitamin. Even normal blood levels, blood levels that are on the low side of normal, can be associated with serious health problems in the form of strokes and heart attacks. Some studies suggest these deficiencies may also be associated with dementia. For these reasons, I recommend supplements of about 400 mcg a day.

"About 5% of us will also develop a deficiency in B12 as we get older. Vitamin B12 deficiency can lead to anemia and serious nerve damage; and so I recommend that you take about 25 to 50 micrograms a day. This is also the amount that is found in most multivitamin preparations.

"As an aside, folic acid might mask the anemia caused by B12 deficiency, but it won't prevent the nerve damage. That's why you shouldn't take folic acid without taking B12. Again, they're neatly combined in many multivitamins at your drugstore."

"Doc, Leonard Johnson again. Next week my son is coming home from medical school for the Christmas break. I want to show him how smart I am. You said something about strokes and heart attacks. Tell us how this folic acid you're talking about could affect strokes."

Homocysteine and vitamin B6

"We'll give it a try, Leonard. For quite some time now, doctors have been aware of an increase in the risk for heart attacks and strokes in people who have an elevated level of a certain amino acid. This amino acid is called homocysteine. The vascular changes associated with elevated levels in some patients may also account for declining mental abilities.

"Homocysteine levels are higher in men than in women; this increases with age. Higher levels are found in people who smoke, have high blood pressure, have high cholesterol, or don't exercise enough. A rare genetic disorder causing elevated levels of homocysteine is associated with severe vascular disease in children. All of this evidence seems to indicate that elevated levels of homocysteine are not good.

"Vitamin B6 and folic acid can help prevent elevated homocysteine levels. Vitamin B6 is also believed to help our immune system fight disease. We should take note that large studies have shown that people with diets that are high in B6 and folic acid have a decreased risk of heart disease. There's lots of it in chicken and fish and to lesser extent in oats, wheat, and nuts. And of course, it's in almost all multivitamin preparations. Garlic is also believed to decrease homocysteine levels; but if you take or eat too much of it, you may become unpopular with your friends.

"Well, we digressed a little and it was fun. Now I want to talk about antioxidants and a little more about vitamins.

Antioxidants

"You remember we discussed those free radical fellows at one of our earlier meetings. Free radicals cause cell damage. They cause us to rust, so to speak, just like free oxygen radicals in the air cause iron to rust. They're called the agents of aging.

"You might recall that they've been linked to many diseases like cancer, cardiovascular disease, cataracts, maybe even wrinkles, and a host of other degenerative things. Our natural defense against these culprits appears to weaken with advancing age, stress, and disease. But there's good news tonight. Certain vitamin and mineral supplements can act as weapons against these free radicals. These free radical 'vacuum cleaners' are called antioxidants.

Vitamin A, beta-carotene and lycopenes

"So now, we'll talk about vitamin A again and also its precursor, beta-carotene. These are antioxidants and seem to be very important for our immune system and our vision. Beta-carotene is converted to vitamin A by your body metabolism. That's why it's called a precursor to vitamin A and is sometimes referred to as pro-vitamin A. Carrots, dark leafy vegetables and fish are excellent sources of beta-carotene or vitamin A as are eggs, whole milk and liver. But you do have to be concerned about the cholesterol and saturated fat in this latter group of foods.

"We've talked about vitamin A toxicity; but you are unlikely to get it from foods that are rich in beta-carotene because the ability of your metabolism to convert beta-carotene to vitamin A is limited. While the habitual and excessive ingestion of carrots or carrot juice can impart a yellow discoloration to the skin, it's a benign condition that disappears when you stop the excess. A similarly, but much less common, benign condition can develop from a chronic overindulgence in tomatoes. Tomatoes contain a pigmented substance called lycopene, another valuable antioxidant. But don't let this information prevent you from eating carrots and tomatoes. They're very healthful. Besides, you would have to eat many, many carrots and tomatoes for these conditions to develop and the discoloration would disappear when you stop the excess. That said, I believe some multivitamin preparations contain a little too much vitamin A. Once again, read the labels and try to take between 2000 IU and 2800 IU a day (0.7 mg for women and 0.9 mg for men).

Vitamin C

"Vitamin C, also known as ascorbic acid, is another important antioxidant. Severe deficiency causes scurvy. Milder deficiency has been linked to a variety of other conditions: heart disease, easy bruising, poor wound healing, cancer, and memory loss. However, the support for this is not definitive and even less so for the belief that vitamin C can prevent colds or other viral illnesses. As previously discussed, taking too much might be harmful. For those of you that think you must take an additional supplement, I don't think you should take more than 250 mg a day.

Multivitamin preparations usually contain 60 mg which is 100% of your recommended daily allowance (RDA); and you get plenty of it from eating citrus fruits, tomatoes, potatoes, and berries. How about that folks? We keep hearing about vegetables, nuts, and fruit. These foods must really be good for us.

Vitamin E

"Green leafy vegetables, nuts, vegetable oils, and wheat germ are all good food sources of vitamin E, which is another antioxidant. There appears to be good evidence that vitamin E is of benefit in promoting cardiovascular health, strengthening the immune system, and possibly even improving prostate health; but the right amount to take each day is controversial. While toxicity is an unlikely event, some studies suggest that taking more than 800 International Units (IU) a day does not appear to produce results that are as good as taking 200 IU to 400 IU a day.

"Now in most instances, the difference between natural and synthetic vitamin preparations is unimportant; but this may not be the case here. Vitamin E is also known as *tocopherol*, of which there are different kinds. Synthetic vitamin E consists almost entirely of alpha-tocopherol whereas natural vitamin E has a mix of alpha, gamma, and delta-tocopherols. Recent studies suggest that the gamma-tocopherols may play a more important protective role than previously thought. Also, some experts believe that the body may process natural vitamin E better than synthetic E. So check the label carefully and look for a mix of tocopherols. Natural vitamin E is labeled as natural but sometimes things are labeled as natural when they're really not. So if you're still not sure, ask the pharmacist. About 400 IU of natural vitamin E is a good daily supplement.

Selenium

"Chicken, fish, nuts, and vegetables are good sources for a mineral called selenium. Selenium is another important antioxidant. Brazil nuts, tuna fish, and asparagus are particularly rich in this mineral; but it is also found in bread and meat. Many studies have strongly suggested that this mineral-antioxidant has cancer prevention qualities. In areas where there are high levels of selenium in the soil, there appears to be a lower rate of death due to cancer. Other studies have shown a decrease in lung, prostate, and colon cancer in people taking a supplement of 200 micrograms a day.

"Most multivitamin preparations contain about 20 micrograms of selenium. If further scientific studies confirm the value of larger amounts, it is likely that future multivitamin preparations will be produced with the appropriate amount. Until then, take your multivitamins and enjoy a healthy intake of fish, vegetables, poultry, and nuts; but be aware of the calories in nuts. As I said, Brazil nuts are particularly high in selenium—but don't get too nuts about nuts."

Fat-soluble vitamins

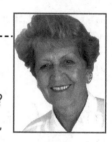

"Dr. Zinney, what do doctors and people mean when they talk about fat-soluble vitamins? What are they?" asked Miriam.

"Fat-soluble vitamins are simply vitamins that are soluble in fat. You know, when we talked about soluble and insoluble fiber we said that soluble fiber is fiber that is soluble in water. Well, fat-soluble vitamins are vitamins that are soluble in fat; and because of that, they're easily stored in our fat tissue and also in our liver. Also because they are soluble in fat, they're probably better absorbed after eating a meal that has some fat. That's why many experts believe that it's better to take your vitamins after dinner or at least after breakfast. Many of us take our vitamins before breakfast, and perhaps we're not absorbing all that we could."

"Interesting advice, Dr. Zinney, but which vitamins are the fat-soluble vitamins?"

"We've already talked about some of them," said Zinney. "Vitamins A, D, E, and K are the so-called fat-soluble vitamins.

Vitamin K

"I've talked about vitamins A and E; so let me spend a few moments talking about vitamins K. Green leafy vegetables are a good source of vitamin K. Smaller amounts are found in eggs, meat, and dairy products. Vitamin K plays an important role in our blood-clotting mechanism. The bacteria that are normally present in our colon are important in furnishing our vitamin K requirements. It is not added to multivitamin tablets because deficiency in this vitamin is extremely rare, except when caused by certain antibiotics. In this uncommon situation, your doctor might prescribe a brief course of treatment with a vitamin K supplement.

Vitamin D

"Vitamin D is quite another story. Milk, butter, eggs, fortified cereals, and seafood are good food sources of vitamin D. Exposure to the sun helps our body actually produce vitamin D. However, we're also told that exposure to the sun is largely responsible for skin aging, skin cancer, and melanomas. Because of this, many experts on the subject urge us to limit our exposure to the sun. If this is coupled with a poor dietary intake, vitamin D deficiency can develop. This sequence of events is common in people who are institutionalized or homebound.

"The importance of vitamin D is that it increases the utilization and absorption of calcium. As we will discover in our next session, this is extremely important in making and maintaining strong bones and in decreasing age-related bone loss. In the past, we believed that 400 IU of vitamin D was the appropriate daily requirement. However, recent studies have shown that some people have low blood levels despite that intake and that bone fractures are more common in those people. Because of these findings, most doctors have come to recommend that the daily intake of vitamin D be increased to 700 or even 800 International Units a day. Most multivitamin pills have about 400 IU in each pill and many supplemental calcium pills have vitamin D added to them. You should really check the label. Women and older men need about 1200 milligrams of calcium a day and most diets only have about 700 milligrams to 800 milligrams a day, so supplements of vitamin D and calcium are important."

"If we don't drink enough milk or eat the other foods that are high in calcium and vitamin D or if we don't take a supplement, will we get osteoporosis?" asked Miriam.

"That's a whole other subject," said Zinney. "But you're partially correct. I had planned to discuss iron, zinc, calcium, and also osteoporosis today; but we're out of time again. So next week we'll talk a little bit about iron and zinc and a whole lot about calcium and osteoporosis. AND I promise, in a few weeks, we'll start on exercise programs and start taking field trips. We had a very interesting evening tonight. Thank you for coming. I look forward to seeing all of you next week."

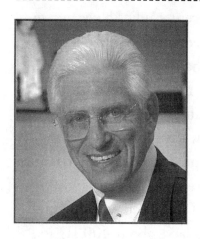

Fiber Content of Selected Foods

Item	Size/Serving	Soluble Fiber Content per serving	Insoluble Fiber Content per serving	Fiber Content per Serving
FRUITS & NUTS				
Almonds (roasted)	1/2 cup	0.78	7.17	7.95
Apple, (with peel)	1 medium	0.97	1.79	2.76
Apricots	1 cup	1.25	2.18	3.13
Banana	1 medium	0.64	1.55	2.19
Cantaloupe	1 wedge	0.64	0.43	1.07
Grapefruit	1 medium	2.21	1.4	3.61
Grapes	1 cup	0.34	0.78	1.12
Orange	1 medium	1.9	1.19	3.14
Peanuts	1/2 cup	2.38	3.96	6.34
Pear, (with peel)	1 medium	1	3.32	4.32
Plums	1 medium	0.66	0.33	0.99
Prunes, (canned)	1 cup	7.88	5.88	13.76
Raspberries	1 cup	0.49	5.79	6.03
Strawberries	1 cup	1.04	2.83	3.87
Walnuts	1/4 cup	1.4	0.9	0.5
Watermelon	1 slice	0.96	0.96	1.93
BREAD, CEREALS & OTHERS				
bran	1 ounce	1.45	7.27	8.72
brown rice	1/2 cup	0.37	4.9	5.27
corn flakes	1 ounce	0.1	0.35	0.45
oat bran	1 ounce	2.04	2.13	4.08
oatmeal	1 ounce	1	1.5	2.51
rye	1 slice	0.36	1.35	1.72
shredded wheat	1 ounce	0.45	2.18	2.64
Spaghetti	2 ounces	1.47	1.09	2.56
white	1 slice	0.24	0.25	0.5
white rice	1/2 cup	0.31	1.11	1.42
whole wheat	1 slice	0.46	1.65	2.11
VEGETABLES				
Asparagus	1/2 cup	0.31	1.17	1.48
Broccoli	1/2 cup	1.15	1.42	2.58
Brussels Sprouts	1/2 cup	1.41	2.09	3.51
Cabbage, green	1/2 cup	0.56	0.95	1.5
Carrots	1/2 cup	0.94	1.48	2.42
Cauliflower	1/2 cup	0.77	1.54	2.3
Celery, (raw)	1/2 cup	0.42	0.54	0.96
Corn	1/2 cup	1.31	1.72	3.03
Cucumber	1/2 cup	0.1	0.42	0.52
Green Peas	1/2 cup	0.48	3.04	3.36
green/string canned	1/2 cup	0.46	1.43	1.89
kidney beans	1/2 cup	1.38	4.1	5.48
Lettuce, iceberg (raw)	1/2 cup	0.06	0.19	0.24
lima beans	1/2 cup	0.85	3.57	4.25
Onions,(raw)	1/2 cup	0.64	0.64	1.28
pinto beans	1/2 cup	1.86	4.09	5.93
Potato (baked w/skin)	1/2 cup	0.7	0.78	1.95
Spinach	1/2 cup	0.47	1.61	2.07
Tomato(raw)	1/2 cup	0.45	0.72	1.17
white beans	1/2 cup	1.06	3.67	4.72

8

Minerals, Hormones, Skin, and Bones

Try your best
To tie the suture
That makes your nest
A better future.

"SURPRISE!" A chorus of voices rang out and sang "Happy Birthday" to Zinney. The discussion group had learned of Zinney's birthday and conspired with Martha to get to the community center early and surprise him with a party of carrot cake and a few bottles of Chardonnay and Cabernet. Zinney was genuinely delighted; and after shyly saying thank you several times, he suggested that they begin the evening's discussion.

"Wait a minute, Doc. Before we begin, how about a speech—or at least tell us how old you are today," Sam asked.

"Well, first I'll tell you how old I am; then I'll start a speech on minerals and other supplements. Today is my sixty-ninth birthday, and I can't remember ever being more delightfully surprised."

"Sixty-nine. You're sixty-nine? That means you're middle aged, at least in this group. Half the people here are younger than you and the other half are older," laughed Craig. "Now you can use those new special slot machines in Las Vegas, special for seniors."

"What kind of slot machines do you mean?" asked Zinney.

"Well, if you get three prunes, you get to go to the crap table," Craig chuckled.

"That's cute," Zinney replied. "Vegas is becoming a very popular place for retirement. So much so that it's changing from the land of Milk and

Honey into the land of Milk of Magnesia. Now if we're about done with our 'drunken debauchery' let's have fun with tonight's discussion."

Menu additions

"Come on Doc, you don't think a little wine will hurt us," asked Leonard.

"As a matter of fact it may actually help us guys," Zinney replied. "But women and men appear to metabolize alcohol differently. Some recent data seems to indicate that the daily ingestion of a couple of alcoholic drinks in women may be associated with some hazards, like an increase in the incidence of breast cancer. But don't panic, ladies. More information is in the making. That said, you'll probably be pleased to know that studies in men suggest that one or two alcoholic drinks a day, particularly red wine, is good for your heart and may actually be associated with greater longevity.

"For both men and women, however, this also appears to be the case for tea and chocolate, particularly dark chocolate. That's good news for all you tea drinkers and chocoholics."

"Hey that's great!" sparked Kinder. "Now my wife can't complain about my wine anymore."

"Well now, John, remember, I said one or two glasses of wine. By that I mean wine glasses not tumblers or bottles," said Zinney.

"Some additional points of interest: there's now some scientific reasons to believe that fish, walnuts, asparagus and berries, particularly blueberries, can improve or help preserve brain function. For example: mice that were fed blueberries dramatically improved their ability to negotiate a maze. While I suspect there's some truth to these scientific stories, the jury is still out. But it's really interesting, isn't it. Mom always said that fish was a brain food and now there's some scientific evidence suggesting that the blueberry is too.

"Dr. Zinney, I want to make sure I've got you straight on this stuff," said Miriam. "You're telling us that nuts, chocolate and tea are good for us? And also, I'd like to know how often you think we should eat fish?"

"As you know, fish is a great source of protein; and as you will recall, fish contain those wonderful omega 3 oils, great antioxidants. You should try to eat fish at least two or three times a week. And it seems that the polyphenols in tea and some of these other foods have multiple beneficial effects. I don't think you should eat the same thing everyday. I think you should vary your foods; but eating a little chocolate, drinking a couple of cups of tea and having some nuts most days seems like a pleasant and healthful idea. As an example, peanuts are also good. Some studies, in women, suggest that eating a handful of peanuts or eating peanut butter a few times a week can significantly reduce the incidence of adult onset diabetes.

"Anyway, we've previously extolled the healthful merits of most of these foods; and I've digressed too much already. Many of you have indicated enormous enthusiasm to hear something about hormones and Retin-A. So before discussing some of the important minerals, we'll take on what tickles your fancy first; and we'll start with estrogen for the 'people from Venus'.

Estrogen

"After the onset of menopause, estrogen replacement, by pills or patches, retards the progression of osteoporosis, or softening of the bones. This is really important because it can decrease bone fractures, bone pain, and shrinking height. You know how some ladies feel when they get older—they're only half the girl they used to be.

"Many women who take estrogen replacement therapy have noted a dramatic improvement in their sense of well being and their quality of life. These effects range anywhere from control of hot flashes and unbearable night sweats to improved sexuality, smoother skin, and better vaginal lubrication. For these reasons, estrogen replacement seems to have an anti-aging effect.

"Estrogen also appears to have a positive effect on the brain by encouraging the growth of brain cells and improving their chemical activity. Whether or not it has any effect on people with Alzheimer's disease is unclear. Some studies have indicated an improvement in memory but others have failed to confirm these findings. We'll have to await the results of additional research while the stew still simmers.

"Despite all these wonderful benefits, estrogen therapy is not without risks. Recent research has shown that the risk of developing breast cancer, uterine cancer, heart attacks, and strokes is increased in some women while taking estrogen and progesterone as hormone replacement therapy [HRT] for menopause. These studies are ongoing in women taking estrogen alone, without progesterone. While the jury is still out on that branch of the study, the result may suggest similar risks.

This could be of particular importance to those who have a strong family history of these problems; the risks may outweigh the benefits. Like so many other things in life, each of us has to weigh the risk-to-benefit ratio of doing something or not doing it—or taking something or not taking it. So, the decision as to whether or not to take estrogen should be individualized and thoroughly discussed with your doctor.

Testosterone

"Now for the bulls, or the 'people from Mars,' we'll talk about testosterone, also known as the male sex hormone. The male climacteric is the male counterpart of the female menopause; but generally, it occurs more gradually. During this change, there is a gradual decline in the production of this sex hormone along with a corresponding decline in libido and sexual performance. When testosterone is given to castrated men, there is a marked improvement in muscle size and strength and, in some cases, an improvement in sexuality. However, in normal men the effects are less consistent.

"Testosterone does not appear to improve impotence in most men. It appears that impotency is related less to testosterone deficiency than to the presence of other problems such as vascular disease, diabetes, and psychological factors like depression. Additionally, the frequency of these problems increases as we age; and many of the medications used to treat them can decrease libido and sexual performance.

"Testosterone is an androgenic steroid that builds protein and muscle; but taking it has some serious potential downside. It may provoke or enhance the growth of prostate cancer. It may encourage the development of coronary artery disease, liver disease, or even male baldness and the growth of facial hair. It's probably not as hazardous as some of the other anabolic-androgenic type steroids that some athletes take. You've all heard horror stories about otherwise healthy people getting liver disease, liver cancer, premature heart disease, and more from anabolic steroids. Some steroids do have some medical uses; but, PLEASE don't take them unless advised by your doctor for a specific reason.

"There's a great deal of research on testosterone therapy and its ability to improve muscle and bone strength. Hopefully, some answers as to its anti-aging effects will become clearer soon. Until then, be patient and take testosterone only for specific reasons under your physician's care. Now let's talk a little about DHEA.

DHEA

"If you are taking DHEA, I would suggest you stop until you consult your doctor. The letters stand for a long chemical name—dehydroepiandrosterone, but no one should expect you to remember that. Health food stores throughout the country have promoted DHEA as a virtual fountain of youth. This substance is a hormone that's normally produced by the adrenal glands and is then converted in your body into estrogen and testosterone. It's been touted as the answer to a multitude of aging problems from preventing cancer, osteoporosis, diabetes, and cardiovascular disease to improving sexual performance and immune systems. Some people have promoted it as an anti-dementia substance. Although DHEA may in fact have some health benefits for certain individuals, taking it can be risky. Additional animal research and then some good human research is needed to determine the real benefits, risks, side effects, and proper dosages of DHEA before I would recommend it. If it is good for some people, we don't yet know who it's good for and who it's not good for. And, we don't know for certain how much you should take."

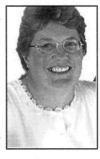

"I've taken some DHEA," said Bertha. "If it's naturally made by our adrenal glands, what's the problem with taking it?"

"As I said, DHEA is converted in our body to estrogen and testosterone; but the proportions are not predictable. That means that someone might get too much estrogen and someone else might get too much testosterone. So this might cause baldness and the growth of facial hair in some women and feminization in some men. More importantly, it may encourage the growth of breast, uterine, or prostate cancer. It might even change blood lipids and encourage the development of heart disease."

"If it's naturally made in our adrenal glands, why would anyone even think we need to take it anyway?" asked Leonard.

"Good question again, Leonard," Zinney responded. "The production of DHEA by our adrenal glands does decrease as we get older. The proponents of the drug suggest that by taking it we can increase our blood levels to what they are in younger adults. The truth is, we can't be sure what those amounts really are. The FDA hasn't approved this stuff for anything.

More research is needed. We should wait until the results are in before we buy into all the hype.

Human Growth Hormone

"Human growth hormone (HGH) and a substance called insulin-like growth factor have been suggested as anti-aging agents," Zinney continued. "Several studies have shown an increase in muscle mass and bone strength in older men and women given HGH. However, long-term follow up studies revealed that the benefits were not maintained. Some of the benefits achieved actually reversed after a period of time.

"Some scientists think that HGH stimulates the production of *insulin-like growth factor* and that the insulin-like growth factor may actually be responsible for the observed benefits. Additional research is in progress to see if any real and sustainable anti-aging benefits can occur by giving either HGH and or insulin-like growth factor to the elderly. If the research shows that the major benefits are derived from insulin-like growth factor and if the cost and side effects of it are minimal, it could be a huge anti-aging boon. Until we know more, the potential side effects and the cost of treatment with HGH are such that I would not recommend it."

"It seems you're always scaring us about side effects, Dr. Zinney," said Leonard. "What are the side effects? And where does this HGH come from?"

"Well, Leonard, I'm just telling you the truth," Zinney replied. "I wouldn't take it myself until I knew more about it. Human growth hormone is made by the pituitary gland. An excess of this hormone in childhood can cause tremendous growth and abnormal height, a condition called *giantism.* Some of the people afflicted with this condition have become famous circus performers, unkindly referred to as freaks. The excess production of this hormone is usually the result of a glandular tumor or over activity of the pituitary gland. When this occurs in adults, it can produce a condition called *acromegaly.* A very famous heavyweight boxing champion, Primo Carnera, suffered from this condition. It's associated with unusually large hands, distortion of facial features, and other abnormalities that lead to high blood pressure, a tendency to develop diabetes and early death. So you see, I think we should learn more about HGH before going across the ocean or south of the border to get this kind of treatment."

Melatonin

"Dr. Zinney, I've been taking melatonin to help me sleep," said Sheila. "Is there any danger to that?"

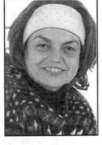

"If you don't take too much of it, it's probably safe. But I don't think we can be positive yet. I'm sure many of you have heard of melatonin. It's a hormone produced in the pineal gland. This little gland is deep inside the brain, as shown on this slide [fig. 8A].

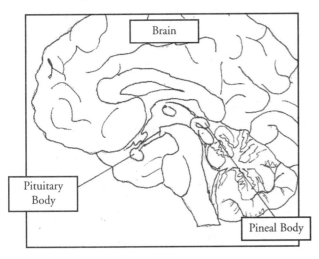

Fig 8A

"The hormone melatonin appears to have antioxidant properties and may also strengthen the immune system. Higher levels are produced at night. This is one reason it is believed to be important in helping us sleep. The elderly have lower levels of melatonin than young adults. These low levels have been linked to the insomnia that occasions advancing age.

"Many travelers have touted it as a cure for jet lag. Others have advocated it as a sleep remedy. Small doses of 0.1 milligrams to 0.3 milligrams have been shown to shorten the time required to fall asleep and to improve the quality of sleep in some individuals. But larger amounts have been associated with headaches and drowsiness during the day.

"Melatonin doesn't require a prescription. The dose commonly sold in stores can be as high as 3 milligrams—many times the amount that appears to be needed. However, a recent study done on blind patients started with doses as high as 10 milligrams a day. These folks live without many of the external environmental factors that influence sleep. Starting with this high dose, many of the patients did experience a restoration of their normal sleep rhythm and even maintained it when the dose was gradually reduced to 0.5 milligrams per day. The timing of the dose was individualized to each patient as determined by blood tests that measured their levels of melatonin. I don't think taking it in small amounts like 1 milligram once in awhile on an intermit-

123

tent basis will be harmful; but I can't recommend it as a daily or regular supplement until we have more solid data. And I wouldn't recommend it in high doses except under the supervision of a physician.

"Now, are there anymore questions on hormones? I don't see any raised hands, so I guess there are none. Ok then, let's start talking about calcium, iron, and other minerals.

Calcium

"Calcium, along with vitamin D, is extremely important to bone health. I'm sure you will recall our prior discussion on the important role that vitamin D plays in the utilization of calcium. Dairy products, foods fortified with calcium, and vegetables like broccoli and kale are rich dietary sources of calcium. Older adults need about 1200 mg. to 1600 mg. of calcium and about 700 IU to 800 IU [international units] of vitamin D daily. In many instances, we only get about 700 mg. of calcium and an insufficient amount of vitamin D. So taking calcium with vitamin D supplements is a good way to slow or help prevent the bone loss that accompanies osteoporosis. Tablets containing 500 mg. to 600 mg. of calcium with 400 IU of vitamin D are available

without a prescription. Since vitamin D is a fat soluble vitamin, better absorption and utilization might be achieved by taking one tablet after breakfast and one after dinner."

"Doc, you got us so sensitized to side effects, I've got to ask you, are there any dangers to taking too much calcium?" Craig asked.

"Glad you asked that question," Zinney responded. "The answer is yes—for some people. There are people who have a tendency to form calcium kidney stones, some of whom might have their condition worsened by taking calcium. There are also people who have an uncommon hormone problem known as hyperparathyroidism and also people that have certain kinds of cancer that can elevate the level of blood calcium. That's why I've emphasized over and over again that your doctor should be aware of all of your supplements."

"I can't get my doctor to spend the time to go over that stuff," Craig said.

"Sure you can," replied Zinney. "Doctors know that your diet and any supplements you're taking are just as important as your medications. They'll take the time to go over this with you just like they'll go over your medications with you."

"Not my doctor," Craig retorted.

"I hope you're wrong, Craig. Your family doctor or a designated assistant should advise you in regard to supplements and diet. But if your doctor won't, find a family doctor that will," Zinney said.

Osteoporosis

"Dr. Zinney, my doctor told me that he thinks I have osteoporosis; and he suggested that I have some kind of a screening scan," Miriam stated. "I guess this is the same as softening of the bones or thinning of the bones. But what is it? What really happens?"

"Osteoporosis or a loss of bone mass and bone mineral density affects both men and women. It starts earlier and is more severe in women. That's why when we get older, many of us will get shorter and suffer serious fractures. Falls and fractures are actually a greater risk factor than obesity in the elderly. As an example: in the USA, there's about 30,000 to 35,000 deaths related to hip fractures each year and more than 20,000 of them occur in post-menopausal women. This can give you some idea of the devastating consequences of osteoporosis.

The make up of bone

"I think it would prove helpful to have some understanding of the anatomy or the make up of bone to more fully appreciate the process. Let's begin there and we'll use a big bone like the femur or thigh-bone as an example for this discussion. As you can see from this diagram [fig. 8B], there is an outer portion of the bone called cortical bone and the inner or more central part of the bone called the matrix. This is also known as cancellous or trabecular bone. The cortical bone is more or less solid and the matrix or trabecular bone is sort of a honeycombed network of bone.

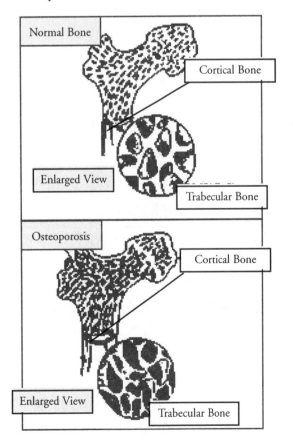

Fig 8B

Bone remodeling and resorption

"The remodeling of bone is a constant and very exciting process. By 'remodeling' I mean that bone is in a constant state of flux. While new bone is being made, old bone is being taken away—a process called resorption.

"This process of bone remodeling—production and resorption, continues throughout our lives. Now—new bone production occurs at a much more rapid rate than bone resorption during our years of growth. When we reach the age of 30 or 35, bone mass reaches its maximum. The rate of production and the rate of resorption seems to remain equal until we are about 40 or 50 years of age. After that, there is a slow loss in the mass of cortical bone in both men and women. Loss of trabecular bone begins slightly earlier in both sexes and is of greater magnitude in women.

"When the rate of bone resorption exceeds the rate of bone production, our bone mass begins to decrease. The rate of bone loss can dramatically accelerate in women around the time of menopause and can be as high as 40 to 50 percent. Although the rate of bone loss is less in men, it can still be quite serious, as high as 20 to 30 percent. We're talking about major losses here. We're talking about getting smaller and becoming fragile. That's why there's

some truth to the song: 'I'm only half the man I used to be.' "

"Does what you're describing occur all over our skeletons?" asked Leonard.

"Yes, but more so in some bones than in others," Zinney answered. "The spine and hips of both men and women and the wrists of women are usually the bones that show the greatest bone loss, and it's mostly a loss in trabecular bone. This correlates with what you already know: we get into the most trouble with fractures and pain in our hips, wrists, and our backs. Vertebral bone fractures—you know those little bones that make up our spine, are usually compression fractures. They can cause a loss of height or even alter the curvature of our spine."

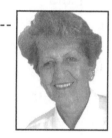

"This sounds terrible," Miriam said. "Is this unstoppable? How or why does this happen? There must be something we can do about it."

"There is Miriam," said Zinney. "Let's talk a little more about how it happens so that we might have a better understanding of how to prevent or slow this process down," Zinney said. "You already know that as the process of bone resorption accelerates we can get what is commonly referred to as softening or thinning of the bones or more appropriately called osteoporosis. Now, the agents of bone production are little cells known as osteoblasts (bone makers) and the agents of bone resorption are little cells known as osteoclasts (bone takers). Since the remodeling of bone is a continuing process throughout our lives, both the osteoblasts and the osteoclasts serve important functions. The osteoblast cells produce new bone and the osteoclast cells resorb bone [fig. 8C].

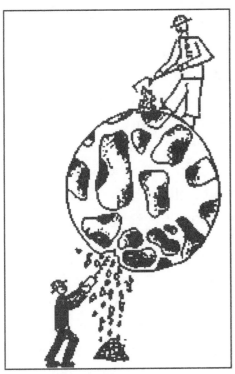

Fig 8C

"Osteoblasts are extremely active during our stages of growth and at the site of fractures, producing new bone to heal the fracture. With advancing age, the activity of the osteoclasts, the agents of bone resorption, exceed the activity of the osteoblasts.

Treatment and prevention

"So now we have a situation of bone makers against bone takers. What we have to do is stimulate or assist the friendly osteoblasts to get on with their work of producing bone and discourage those nasty little osteoclasts from taking bone away from us. To do this, we have to give our friendly osteoblasts the tools to win. The most important tools are calcium, vitamin D, exercise, bone sparing medications and in selected cases, estrogen (in women) and testosterone (in some men). We've already discussed the importance of vitamin D, calcium, and hormones; but I can't emphasize the importance of exercise strongly enough. We'll talk more about this a little later.

"Diets that are deficient in calcium or vitamin D, or intestinal disorders and liver disease that impair the absorption of calcium, are associated with accelerated bone loss. Cigarette smoking or too much vitamin A and estrogen deficiency in women as well as testosterone deficiency in men, increases the risk of bone loss and osteoporosis. Recent research also suggests that women who drink more than three cups of coffee a day may increase their risk of bone loss. People who are immobilized due to illness and people who lead a sedentary life, as in the case of couch potatoes, also suffer a pronounced loss of bone. But exercise, stressing your bones with resistance training, can dramatically enhance the activity of our friendly osteoblasts.

Resistance training and osteoporosis

"In this regard, weightlifting exercises and other types of resistance training can be extremely important. In one study, the bone density of the femoral neck, where so many fractures occur, was increased by 3.8% after just 16 weeks of training. In another study that involved post-menopausal women from 50 to 70 years old, the bone mineral density of the lumbar spine was increased by 6.3% after one year of training. The control group that was not involved in the training program, experienced a loss of bone mineral density of 3.7% during the same period of time. This amounted to a real difference of 10% between those who were in training and those who did not train. Other studies have shown similar results, even in women who are not taking estrogen. Strong muscles are associated with strong bones. Strengthening our muscles will strengthen our bones. But it's important to appreciate that retarding the progress or even preventing severe osteoporosis with these measures is far

easier and more effective than treating advanced osteoporosis after it's become established."

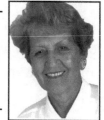

"Well, what good is my getting that scan if we can't treat it?" asked Miriam.

Bone sparing medications

"I didn't say that we can't treat osteoporosis. We can treat it, Miriam; but it's easier to prevent than to treat. Exercise, calcium, vitamin D, and hormone replacement therapy, if recommended by your doctor, are very effective measures that can retard the progress of osteoporosis. Once it has developed, these same measures, combined with the use of certain medications can be effective in treating the condition.

"In established osteoporosis, a hormone called *calcitonin* can be taken by nasal spray along with calcium supplements. This hormone can increase bone density and prevent fractures. An even more effective group of medicines known as *biphosphonates* (Didronel and Fosamax) can be used. These drugs, when taken with calcium and vitamin D, can increase bone density and bone strength. They've been shown to decrease fractures of the wrist and hip. They work by decreasing the activity of the osteo-clasts, the little buggers that take bone away.

"More recently, a medication called *Evista* (raloxofene) has shown very promising results in treating osteo-porosis. Its effects are similar to estro-gen on bone production and the pre-vention of bone loss; but its effects are anti-estrogen on breast and uterine tis-sue. So, as it improves bone mineral density, it may also protect against breast cancer. As an important word of caution, keep in mind that these drugs are prescription medications. They all have significant side effects and should only be taken under care-ful medical supervision.

"There's yet another interesting devel-opment on the horizon. Observational studies suggest that a class of medica-tion known as *statins*, which are used to treat high cholesterol, may have a beneficial effect on bone density. It seems that they might also inhibit the action of osteoclasts. Patients taking this medication appear to have a much lower incidence of fractures and greater degree of bone mineral density. While there is much research to be done on this subject, we can all be hopeful. These statins have compara-tively few side effects; and they, or some pharmacological modification of them, could be a boon to the treat-ment and the prevention of osteo-porosis in the future.

DEXA scan

"Now, Miriam, in terms of the scan you asked about. I assume your doctor wants you to have what is commonly called a DEXA scan."

"Yes. That's it, Dr. Zinney. But maybe you could tell me what that is," said Miriam.

"Sure," said Zinney. "The term DEXA is short for Dual Energy X-ray Absorptiometry. This painless test does not expose you to high levels of radiation. It's far more effective than conventional x-rays in determining bone density and diagnosing osteo-porosis. As a screening procedure, peripheral scans rather than total body scans can be performed. These are scans done on the ankles or wrists. If osteoporosis is detected, then a total body scan can be performed to deter-mine the severity and extent of the osteoporosis. Remember, if the scan shows that you already have osteo-porosis, you can still benefit from the preventative and therapeutic measures we've discussed."

Osteoarthritis

"Is osteoporosis the same as osteoarthritis?" asked Bertha.

"No. They can be easily confused because they are both very common. Both begin at about the same age, both involve bones and joints, and both start with *osteo*. However, they are two very different animals," replied Zinney. "Osteoarthritis usually involves the fingers, knees, hips, shoulders, and spine. Symptoms can begin as early as the third decade and are common by the age of forty.

"By the age of seventy, almost everybody has developed some osteoarthritis. For this reason, it has been commonly referred to as degenerative arthritis. This term serves to clearly differentiate it from inflammatory diseases like rheumatoid arthritis, the other arthritis with which it is often confused. Let's be clear. Osteoarthritis bears no relationship to rheumatoid arthritis or similar inflammatory diseases.

"With the wear and tear of time, the cartilage that cushions our joints becomes roughened and pitted and begins to decrease in size; it begins to degenerate. This results in a grating of the bones that make up our joints. The added stress and irritation of the bony surfaces of the joints stimulates the bone to grow bone spurs and osteophytes, fragments of bone often referred to as joint mice. Interestingly, this disease is not limited to human beings. It would appear that osteoarthritis actually evolved along with the vertebrate skeleton because it has been found in prehistoric dinosaurs, whales, fish, and birds.

"While osteoarthritis is usually a slow progressive disorder, it can stop or even reverse. The onset of pain is gradual. At first, morning stiffness usually decreases with fifteen to twenty minutes of activity. Limitation of motion, joint swelling, increasing pain with motion, and joint tenderness can become more apparent as the condition progresses.

Treatment

"Various forms of physical therapy (exercise, cold packs, hot packs, massage, acupuncture, etc.) are the mainstay of treatment and have proven to be successful in most cases. Stretching exercises that preserve the range of motion and resistance exercises that help strengthen the muscles and stabilize the joint are very effective. In this regard, back and wrist or knee supports can also be beneficial.

"While drug therapy is the least important aspect of treatment, pain can often be alleviated with Tylenol or muscle relaxants. Aspirin or non-steroidal anti-inflammatory drugs, commonly referred to as NSAIDS or

COX-1 inhibitors (Motrin, Naprosyn, etc.) may be used, but their continued use may have adverse effects.

"NSAIDS can cause kidney damage and may irritate your gastrointestinal tract and cause ulcers and bleeding. However, a new variety of NSAIDS has recently been introduced that works a little differently. They're called COX-2 inhibitors (Celebrex, Vioxx, etc.). They are less likely to cause gastrointestinal irritation, but please be cautious with them because all of these drugs can have serious side effects. So, check with your doctor before using them on a regular basis. Please, try to stay away from strong pain relievers like narcotics and narcotic-like drugs. Habituation, reliance, and addiction are easy to come by and hard to leave behind.

"On a new note, a member of the tetracycline group of antibiotics, known as Doxycycline, seems to slow or even prevent the progression of osteoarthritis. It's believed to work by blocking some of the enzymes that break down cartilage. Extensive research is in progress to determine its effectiveness, but the jury is still out."

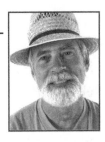

"Doc, I've heard a lot of people are taking some stuff called chondroitin and glucosamine. Can you tell us something about it?" asked John.

"You read my mind, John," Zinney replied. "There have been several reports suggesting that the combination of chondroitin sulfate and glucosamine can be helpful with osteoarthritis. Chondroitin sulfate is an important ingredient in the cartilage and connective tissue of all animals; and the other stuff, glucosamine serves as a building block for many of the constituents that make up joints and joint fluids. In my experience, about twenty-five percent of folks who have early disease feel better taking these agents. You can buy the combination tablet in almost any pharmacy without a prescription. Since I don't know of any toxicity associated with it, I think it's worth a try.

"The injection of cortisone drugs directly into the joint may be helpful when swelling or other signs of inflammation are present. Generally, these drugs are used intermittently and as infrequently as possible. But, on a different note, a substance called Hyaluronic acid, which is a normal constituent of joint fluid, has proved very helpful. Intra-articular injections of commercial preparations of Hyaluronic acid (Hyalgan, ARTZ, Synvisc) have resulted in a measurable and surprisingly sustained improvement in a large number of patients.

Alternative therapy

"While it may not alter the course of the disease, acupuncture has helped many by relieving the pain secondary to osteoarthritis. In this way, it can serve as a valuable adjunct to a good physiotherapy program. However, the claim held by many Naturopaths that specific diets, herbs, and vitamin supplements can successfully treat osteoarthritis is without any scientific proof, and I can't recommend such an endeavor. If you're going to follow that kind of a program, please check with your doctor to make sure he or she knows what you're taking and what you're doing.

"That having been said, a diet can help. It is well known that osteoarthritis can be more severe in obese people because of the added pressure on joints. A diet intended to induce weight reduction in these patients will reduce stress on weight bearing joints. This can help to decrease pain and even slow the progress of the disease.

Surgical treatment

"In the event that conservative therapy fails, the disease often progresses with increasing pain, severe limitation of motion, and a mounting compromise of one's ability to ambulate. This is when surgery can be of enormous value in restoring the quality of life. A minimally invasive procedure, known as arthroscopy, involves the insertion of a special scope into the joint space. Fragments of cartilage and other troublesome debris lining the joint space can be removed. While it is believed to reduce pain, recent studies have questioned its effectiveness. In more advanced situations, an arthroplasty can be performed. It consists of an open surgery to repair the joint and can frequently produce wonderful long-term improvement.

"In even more advanced osteoarthritis, partial or even total joint replacement may be preferable. Complete replacement of knee joints, hip joints, and shoulder joints have been successful in more than ninety percent of cases. However, before undergoing any of these procedures, and particularly before becoming the bionic man, make sure you have an orthopedic surgeon who is experienced in these operations and consider a consultation with a good rheumatologist.

Iron

"If there are no more questions, we can go on. We'll continue our discussion on minerals. Iron is a very important mineral. Meat, vegetables, fortified cereals, and eggs are good nutritional sources of iron. Most of us get all the iron we need from these foods.

"However, many people take lots of iron pills and syrups to improve their energy level or combat fatigue. I'm opposed to that for two reasons. First, it can mask the presence of the development of an iron deficiency problem that may be of a serious nature. Second, iron can accumulate in the liver and cause or worsen liver disease. In many instances, iron deficiency and anemia can be quickly corrected by taking iron. But, that's not only part of the solution, it can also be part of the problem as well. Let me explain.

"Iron is important in making hemoglobin, an essential part of our red blood cells. When these red blood cells are pumped through our lungs, the hemoglobin picks up the oxygen we inhale and carries it to the different parts of our body. That's how the muscles and all of the tissues in our body get oxygen. When we don't have enough iron to make enough hemoglobin, we develop anemia. In other words, we have fewer red blood cells than we should. There are many types

and many causes for anemia; but this kind of anemia is called *iron deficiency anemia*. In iron deficiency anemia, we not only have less red blood cells, but the blood cells are smaller and contain less hemoglobin than they should. Because of this, they can't carry as much oxygen to the muscles and tissues of our body.

"Although iron deficiency and anemia can result from poor nutrition or impaired absorption of iron, more importantly, it can be caused by the loss of iron as a result of chronic blood loss. A number of conditions, from the very benign to the very serious, can be responsible for this. Examples include peptic ulcer disease, colon cancer, colon polyps, hemorrhoids, and excessive menstrual bleeding—just to name a few. Any kind of chronic blood loss can drain our iron stores and cause iron deficiency and anemia. And because the blood loss can be small, an individual might be unaware of it until he or she develops anemia along with the symptoms of weakness and fatigability.

"Iron deficiency anemia is easily diagnosed with a simple blood test. If chronic blood loss is in fact the cause of the iron deficiency anemia, determining the cause and the source of the blood loss becomes very important. And as we said, it can range from very benign and easily treatable conditions to the very serious. So don't take a lot of iron pills or supplements without your doctor's knowledge or recommendation, as it might mask a serious condition."

"Doc, earlier you mentioned zinc," said Leonard. "What about zinc and all those other minerals? They must be important."

Zinc and other minerals

"A host of important minerals and trace elements are part of our body make-up. Examples include selenium and iron, which we've already discussed, and zinc, magnesium, manganese, chromium, molybdenum, and many others. For the most part, deficiencies in these minerals in the United States are extremely rare. We get sufficient amounts in our diet. Green leafy vegetables, fruits, whole grains, and lean meats serve as generous sources of these microelements. Moreover, there's plenty in most multivitamin preparations. So additional supplementation doesn't appear to be necessary and could actually be harmful.

"Leonard specifically mentioned zinc, so we'll talk a little about zinc. Zinc deficiency has been linked to diminished sexual performance, an altered sense of taste, and an altered sense of smell. In the most unusual and extremely rare circumstance of severe zinc deficiency, enlargement of the liver and spleen and the development of anemia have been reported. Note— the daily requirement of zinc is about 15 milligrams. That's the same amount that's present in many multivitamin pills; and as we said, you get plenty in healthful diet. So there's no proven reason to take any more than that.

"Well, that would seem to rap it up for tonight—unless there are any questions."

Chromium

"You mentioned chromium. I heard that chromium is a fat burner and that taking chromium supplements can help someone lose weight and build muscle. Would you please comment on that for us?" asked Leonard.

"I heard the same thing you did, Leonard; but I don't believe it. Studies have shown no difference in weight loss or muscle development between groups taking chromium and those taking a placebo, a sugar pill. As in the case of zinc, there's enough chromium in most multivitamin preparations," Zinney replied. "At the present time, I would not recommend it as an additional supplement unless further research proves it to be beneficial."

Skin

"Dr. Zinney, I know it's getting late; but, before we go tonight, could you comment on some of the popular anti-wrinkle remedies?" asked Sheila.

"We have some time left," said Zinney. "Before I comment on wrinkle remedies, let's talk a little about our aging skin in general. Most of the effects of aging on the skin are more the result of exposure to the sun than to actual aging. Probably the more appropriate term for these changes is photo-aging. These changes include a variety of different colored spots, rough skin, and a loss of elasticity causing sagging and wrinkling.

"Many of the discolored rough spots we get are called keratoses, unkindly referred to as senile keratoses because they appear as we age. Most are benign lesions and they're of no real consequence other than their appearance. But it is essential that they be differentiated from more serious skin lesions like skin cancer or another type of keratoses called actinic keratoses. Some dermatologists consider this type of keratoses to be precancerous or actually cancer.

Skin cancer

"Skin cancer is very common; and sun exposure markedly increases the risk of developing it. While there are many different types of skin cancer, some are much more serious than others. Let me talk about three types that are clearly related to sun exposure. One kind, called basal cell carcinoma, is a locally invasive cancer that rarely spreads and can usually be treated effectively by your doctor or a dermatologist. Another type, called squamous cell carcinoma, can spread if not detected and treated early. Cure rates are also very good for this type of cancer.

"The third type is really dangerous. This kind is called a melanoma. A melanoma usually appears as a nevus or pigmented spot or mole. If not treated early, it can spread to distant parts of the body; and it can be fatal. However, some recent advances in treatment have shown promising results in about one third of patients; and so, hope is on the way. The important thing to remember is this: if a spot on your skin changes in size, changes in color, begins to itch, or concerns you in any other way, please have your doctor take a look at it. Early diagnosis and treatment are the keys to cure.

Sun screen

"Knowing all this, why would anyone want to be a sunbather? Sure, a little bit of sun can be a good way to get vitamin D, but sunbathing or going to tanning parlors for cosmetic reasons is counter-productive. We all baked on the beach when we were kids and young people are still doing it. They're out there on the beach broiling in the sun. This isn't healthy. This is dangerous. This increases the chance of getting skin cancer, wrinkles, crows feet, keratoses, and God knows what else. If you are still doing this, please stop it! And if you know people, young or old, who are still doing it, tell them to stop!

"For some of us, our work or our favorite activity, like golf or tennis, takes us out into the sun. That's ok. But please wear some protective clothing and a brimmed hat to shield you. Also, use a good sunscreen lotion and be sure to cover all the exposed surfaces of your skin adequately. You should do this whenever you spend time outside. Your skin gets exposed even on cloudy days and even while you're riding in your car. Sure, the glass window screens some of the rays out—but not all of them. The regular use of a good protective lotion can not only prevent further photo-aging and decrease your chances of getting skin cancer, but it can actually reverse some of the damage your skin has already suffered. So the first line of defense against developing 'old skin'

and treating some of the changes that occur is protection from the rays of the sun.

Treating wrinkles

"Many of use would like to actually eliminate our wrinkles but it would be at least as good an idea if we prevented some of them in the first place. As previously discussed, this could be accomplished by avoiding or protecting yourself from excessive exposure to the sun and also by not smoking cigarettes. There's little double in my mind that cigarette smoking speeds and exaggerates the development of wrinkles. However, after wrinkles have developed, there are some interesting things that can be done that can lessen their appearance or even get rid of some of them.

"To start with, some of you have asked me about facial massages and mudpacks. I don't believe expensive facial massages or mudpacks do anything but make your face dirty. Nonetheless, it's clear that most of us do like to look good. That's why we comb our hair, shave or wear makeup. While the degree of importance one might place on their own appearance may vary, for many people, looking better or younger has a very positive effect on their self-confidence and self-esteem. Facial treatments and anti-wrinkle remedies have become big business and it's reason enough to touch on the subject."

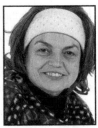

"But how about the creams for wrinkles and spots. Don't some of them work?" asked Sheila.

"The available information suggests that some do. Certain acids like lactic, citric, and particularly glycolic acid, known as 'AHAs' or alpha-hydroxy acids, have been shown to reduce the wrinkling and the thinning of skin that accompanies aging. So far, however, the only 'magic in a bottle' is Retin A cream. When used daily for several months it has reduced small wrinkles and pigmentations. It may also reverse the growth of the previously mentioned precancerous skin condition called actinic keratoses. The longer the use of this cream, the greater benefit. Retin A concentrations of 0.05 percent are more effective than concentrations of 0.02 percent but may cause swelling and redness. However, with continued use, this usually resolves over a period of three to four months.

Plastic surgery

"Redundant skin around your neck, the so-called 'turkey neck;' deep wrinkles, or furrows; sagging jowls; and sagging eyelids cannot be cured with the use of any creams or lotions. The only effective way to alter these changes is with cosmetic surgery, often called reconstructive or plastic surgery. Significant advances have been made in cosmetic surgical techniques so that the discomfort and the recovery time are much less than they used to be. And the results can be very gratifying.

Peels, lasers, and injections

"Chemical peels and some of the newer laser treatments can be very effective in erasing minor wrinkles and reducing furrows. There is swelling and discomfort following any of these procedures; but it usually disappears in two or three weeks.

"Some furrows can be reduced and some wrinkles even erased by injecting collagen directly into a wrinkle or injecting Botox into selected facial muscles. Botox is the pharmaceutical preparation of the food poison that causes botulism. This rare disease can cause fatal paralysis of muscles when food that is contaminated by the bacteria known as Clostridium botulinum is eaten. That said, the pharmaceutical preparation for this popular wrinkle treatment is quite safe in experienced hands. When Botox is injected into selected facial muscles, it relaxes those muscles. This allows many furrows and wrinkles to decrease or even disappear. However, the effects of collagen injections into wrinkles or Botox into facial muscles are not permanent, and the procedure may have to be repeated in three to twelve months.

"The important thing here is, if you are contemplating any of these procedures, be absolutely certain that the surgeon you've selected has good credentials and lots of experience in this type of work. Too much bargain hunting and a failure to investigate can result in catastrophe.

"Whew! We talked about a lot of things tonight and I'm pooped. If there are no more questions, let's call it a night. But remember, the best is yet to come. Next week we'll meet at the YMCA and begin our discussions and demonstrations on exercise, the single most important thing you can do for yourselves. So, have a good week. I look forward to seeing you at our local Y next time."

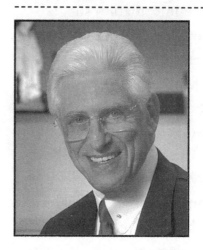

9

On a pound of fat,

Let me make my case—

A pound of muscle,

Takes less space.

About Exercise

By 7:00 P.M. the lecture hall at the Y was only half filled. Joe, the executive director of the Y, sensed Zinney's discomfort and said, "I guess you expected better attendance, but you know, Zinney, you gotta take it in stride. Some days you're the dog, and some days you're the hydrant."

"I'm not really surprised," Zinney replied, "lots of people go to lectures and discussions about fitness and aging because they feel guilty; but only about half of them actually do anything about it. This is particularly true when it comes to exercise. We can talk about all the virtues of exercise tonight but probably only 75 percent will actually start the program; and then, another quarter of them will probably drop out shortly afterwards. The people that get into it and stay with it are the people that will win in the second half. They will be blessed by the natural resources within their own bodies. That's what's uplifting.

Endorphins and enkephalins

"The more people we get involved, the better we'll feel; and more importantly, the better they will feel. You know, Joe, most of us who exercise don't really like to exercise. We only think we like to exercise because we love the way it makes us feel. That's partly because of endorphins. I'm sure you know something about endorphins and enkephalins."

"I've heard of them and know they're supposed to make us feel good when we exercise; but I don't really know what they are," Joe replied.

"Scientifically speaking," Zinney said, "they're called opioid peptides. They're not really related to opium or morphine; but they act at the same receptor sites in our body. The endorphins are produced mostly in our pituitary gland but also in some parts of the brain. That's why it's believed they play an important role in emotions, memory, and learning.

"The enkephalins are produced mostly in our adrenal glands and are released along with other hormones in response to stress. They're all over the body but there are really high levels in the spinal cord and intestinal tract. These natural substances, produced by the body, seem to increase when we exercise. It is believed that the release of endorphins and possibly enkephalins, as well, makes us feel great when we exercise. They're almost addictive. It's probably one of the reasons people who regularly exercise don't feel as well if they miss too many workouts. They miss the invigorating feeling they get from endorphins. They miss the wonderful 'high' and antidepressant effect of their own natural endorphins.

"If we can just get people into it, and keep them going for eight to sixteen weeks, they'll love the way it makes them feel. And they'll keep at it. So let's get started!"

Dr. Zinney began the program by introducing the executive director and his assistants. He explained that they would all be available during and after the program to answer any questions the audience might have regarding the facility and some of the special features it offers.

Why you should exercise

"Friends, I'm particularly glad you brave souls came tonight because you're going to begin what might be the most important journey of the rest of your life, 'The WISH For Fitness Program,'" Zinney said as he paced briskly before the audience while gesturing with a hand-held microphone. "Fitness is not an option, it's an absolute imperative! Together we're going to learn how to improve our strength, our endurance, our balance, and our flexibility.

"Your involvement in an exercise program is not only of major importance to you, it's important to your family and friends. Throughout our previous discussions, we've frequently brushed on the value of exercise. But at this point, even at the risk of being redundant, we will revisit the joy, the value, and the importance of exercise. Regular exercise, at any age, will be a major factor in compressing morbidity. Exercise may or may not enable you to live longer; but it will surely enable you to live better. It's very likely to add years to your life, and it will most certainly add life to your years. That's what I mean by compressing morbidity. You will suffer less illness and you will recover from illnesses more effectively. Of all of the healthful things you can do, regular exercise is probably the singularly most important.

"As an example, some studies have shown that men who smoke cigarettes but who regularly exercise are better off than nonsmokers who don't exercise. Clearly, cigarette smoking is a terrible addiction. I can attest to that on a personal level. Tobacco is not a health food. It is associated with awful diseases and is a major societal health hazard. Anyone who smokes should make every effort to stop; and if they fail once, they should try and try again. Having said that, the suggestion that fitness appears to have an even greater effect on improving longevity and decreasing morbidity further underscores the value of regular exercise. You can have more strength, vigor, vitality, and greater mental clarity.

"No matter how old you are, or how much damage has been done in the first half of your life, or how bad your present conditioning, it's not too late. People who never exercised and begin to exercise between the ages of forty to seventy can get in better shape than the high school and college jocks they knew who gave up exercising. You can make spectacular improvement in your conditioning and the way you feel and look. You will thank your Maker over and over again for the enormous resources preserved in your body—resources that you can call upon at almost any age that will improve your strength and fitness. And you can do this in an amazingly short period of time. You can; you definitely can win in the second half.

"You can become the ambassadors of exercise. Friends and family will be infected by the change in your appearance, the spring in your step, and your increased energy.

"You've taught your children morals and table manners. You taught these things not just by talking, but also by example. Now you must teach them something equally important, even far more important, to their well being and their survival. It doesn't matter how old your kids are now; they still learn from you. You must teach them the value of regular exercise, but you must do so by example. If they're not involved in regular exercise, this is a very important lesson they can learn from you.

"Physical exercise effects more than just muscles and bones. We've previously learned that as the brain ages, there is a decrease in formation of dendrites and synapses, the branching and connecting of our brain and nerve cells. At one time, it was believed that after maturity, the brain had no ability to grow. Now we know differently. Now we know that mental exercise can increase the production of a substance called *brain growth factor* to improve brain function at almost any age. And we've learned that physical exercise actually has a similar effect. It will turn on that amazing computer between our ears and click on all the right symbols.

"Physical exercise increases brain growth factor, increases the blood flow to the brain, increases the branching of the brain cells, and increases the number of synapses, or connections, between them. So, working out regularly has a very positive effect on brain function, particularly as we age. It may not make you smarter but it will improve your brain function so that you can become smarter if you try.

"While improving our muscle and bone strength and our balance, exer-cise also increases good cholesterol and decreases bad cholesterol. It improves our cardiac and lung functions, which can help increase longevity and decrease morbidity. Strength and endurance training also actually improves the functioning of our gastrointestinal tract and our metabolism.

"Strength training, in particular, increases your muscle mass. This increases your metabolic rate, enabling you to burn more calories and fat even at rest. Remember that resting muscle burns more calories than resting fat.

"If you suffer from diabetes, it can improve your sugar metabolism and decrease your insulin requirements. Studies have actually shown increased insulin sensitivity and improved glucose tolerance in people on strength training programs.

What kind of exercise

"Let's talk a little about the importance of strengthening muscles. Between the ages of 40 years and 70 years most men and women will lose about 30 percent to 50 percent of their strength. That's really depressing. But it's not irreversible! This progressive loss of strength is associated with a decrease in muscle mass, a condition called *sarcopenia*. The development of sarcopenia is accelerated by the inactivity that too often accompanies aging; and this can be even further accelerated by chronic disease. Chronic problems like arthritis, emphysema, diabetes, and heart disease can understandably discourage activity and further encourage the development sarcopenia.

"The decrease in muscle strength leads to a decrease in endurance and balance; and this strength-endurance-balance deficit is associated with a decrease in functionality and an increase in falls. Approximately one out of every three seniors will experience a fall each year. As we age, falls and fractures become one of the leading causes of death; and above the age of 85, they are the major cause. Add to this that weak muscles are associated with weak bones (osteoporosis). Osteoporosis is associated with a greater frequency of fractures, more severe fractures, and poor healing of fractures. Strength training, even in elderly people, can improve bone density, muscle strength, and balance. This has the potential to decrease falls and fractures and the grief that can accompany them."

"I think I know, but just exactly what do you mean by strength training?" asked Bertha.

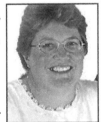

"I mean a form of resistance exercise like weight lifting, weight machines, or pneumatic resistance machines. We'll describe the equipment and how to do the exercises in detail a little later on. The important thing to get is that carefully performed and supervised resistance training can dramatically and quickly strengthen muscles and bones.

"I'm not suggesting that anyone will become an Arnold Schwartzenegger because that's not going to happen. And you women aren't going to become muscular or masculinized amazons either—not unless you want to. Of course, the earlier you start, the better you will be able to prevent osteoporosis. But the benefits are enormous for us old folks as well. Studies show that even if you're between the ages of eighty to ninety you can increase your leg strength by more than 100 percent in just eight to sixteen weeks of supervised training. Walking speed, in the participants of one study, increased by 28 percent and their stair climbing ability increased by 12 percent or more. Some subjects actually threw their walkers and canes away. Not only did their strength improve, but their balance also improved.

"Other studies have shown equally beneficial effects on bone density.

We've discussed some of them previously but I think they warrant additional discussion tonight. The bone density of the neck of the femur (thigh bone) can be increased by 3.8 percent in just 16 weeks of strength training. In a group of post-menopausal women the bone density of the low back (the lumbar spine) was increased by 6.3 percent after just one year of strength training. It should also be noted that the control group of women in this study (the women who did not participate in strength training) lost 3.7 percent of their bone density during this same period of time. That's a total difference of 10 percent in bone density between the women on a strength-training program and the inactive group in just one year. Similarly, upper body strength training will improve upper body strength and bone density. This is all very important because, as I'm sure you know, most fractures in older men and women occur in the hips, wrists, arms, shoulders, and lower spine.

"Do I need to say more? Can you find the time to exercise? The average adult in this country spends about three to four hours a day watching TV or surfing the Internet. Maybe you're an exception and you're not one of these people. You're just too busy and you're just too tired to exercise. That's a bunch of BULL. I don't care how busy you think you are, you have to make the time. We're all familiar with the Surgeon General's warning label on cigarettes. Well I think the Surgeon General should put a warning label on the TV screen of every program that says, 'Watching this program combined with a failure to exercise on a regular basis can accelerate obesity, heart disease, lung disease, diabetes, dementia, osteoporosis, falls, fractures, and death.'"

"That's pretty funny," said Bertha. "But you seemed to be emphasizing strength training. I always thought that cardio-pulmonary exercise was more important."

"By cardiopulmonary training, Bertha is referring to aerobic exercise or endurance training. Of course this is important. A healthy heart and healthy lungs are very, very important. At least 40 percent of us will probably die from some type of cardiovascular disease. Endurance training might cut that risk in half. Yoga, brisk walking, jogging, stair-stepping exercises, and cycling exercises are endurance exercises. And for most of these, all you need is a good pair of shoes.

"But it's really important to realize that strength training and cardiopulmonary training are not enemies of one another. They can be combined. A strength-training program can be configured to give you a good cardiopulmonary workout. Or on the other hand, they can be done on alternate days. They're not mutually exclusive. Stretching exercises to improve flexibility and balance exercises are important also. For greater fitness, they should all be complimentary.

"The different kinds of exercise: strength training, endurance, stretching, and balance training all work together to produce a greater level of fitness. We'll discuss the value of each of them and how to get into them shortly. But you're right, Bertha. I am emphasizing strength training because its importance has been under-appreciated. I can't over-emphasize it. For most of us, it's the key that can unlock the door to better endurance and balance exercises.

"About 15 percent of the seniors in the USA are classified as frail. These frail seniors account for 40 percent to 50 percent of healthcare expenditures. Whether these folks suffer from heart disease, lung disease, arthritis, liver disease, kidney disease, neurological disease, diabetes, or whatever—there's one common denominator to their frailty. It's MUSCLE WEAKNESS! It's sarcopenia. Sure, their primary disease caused their disability and this encouraged further inactivity; but still, each and every one of them share this one feature: MUSCLE WEAKNESS. They fall and even if they don't sustain a fracture they often don't have the strength to get up. Sometimes they quite suddenly find themselves unable to rise from the toilet seat. They become in need of assisted living. They lose most of their independence. Having just discussed some of the relevant studies, we now know that strength training can reverse a lot of this muscle weakness. Not only will strength training prevent many catastrophes, it will help us survive a catastrophe.

"So strength training is an absolute must. We—all of us—have to do it. And later, we're going to learn how to do it the right way. Believe me, once you get started you'll love it. Once you get started, you won't want to live without it.

"Those of us who are in pretty good shape can start an exercise program that combines strength training, stretching exercises, endurance training, and balance exercises at the same time. But many of us can't do this. We can't effectively perform balance and endurance exercises because of a lack of strength. In these instances, improving the individual's strength as a first order of business will better equip them to perform balance and endurance exercises later.

"Strength training can, and should, be combined with stretching exercises to improve flexibility. Both have a very beneficial effect on balance. When special balance exercises are then added, the results can be spectacular. Obviously, weak leg muscles can't effectively perform aerobic exercise like jogging, stair climbing, or even brisk walking. Lower body strength training can prepare the leg muscles for these exercises and further improve their performance. Strength training can even be performed as a cardiopulmonary workout. But as I said, we'll get into all this and the different types of exercises later. I hope I answered your question, Bertha."

"You did, Dr. Zinney but you raised another one in my mind," said Bertha. "Most of us aren't frail like the 15 percent of the seniors you've described. So why should we have to do this?"

"Now, Bertha! You have to remember what we said about losing strength as we get older. You're going to lose between 1 percent and 1.5 percent of your strength each year; and our lower body strength seems to wane more quickly than our upper body strength. This is because we do a lot of sitting. While both are important, serious attention has to be given to our lower body—our legs.

"Even if you don't become frail, you're going to be a lot weaker; and you should note that frailty can descend upon any of us quite suddenly, as a result of illness or an accident. What I need all of you to remember is this: a great deal of the muscle weakness associated with aging can be prevented by strength training; and even more importantly, a great deal of it can be reversed. So we're going to do it."

Aerobic and anaerobic exercise

"But everybody seems to stress the importance of aerobic exercise for your heart and lungs. You stress strength training. I'm confused," said Sam. "Will 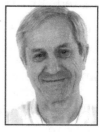 strength training also benefit our heart? And doesn't aerobic exercise burn more calories than strength training? What's the difference between the two?"

"Good question, or should I say, questions," Zinney replied. "First let me say that aerobic exercise is endurance training; or some refer to it as cardiopulmonary conditioning. Aerobic exercise, like brisk walking, is extremely important to the health of your heart and lungs. It will be an essential part of the exercise program we'll teach you. Strength training, building muscles, is an important part of increasing endurance. And it can benefit both your heart and lungs also. We need to do both aerobic exercise and strength training.

Muscle physiology

"To appreciate this more, it might help to understand a little muscle physiology, and to learn how the muscle cell produces and utilizes energy. As our muscles exercise, they utilize energy and produce a chemical called lactic acid, or lactate. Muscle lactate is the metabolic end-product of the exercising muscle. The oxygen that we breathe is carried by our blood to the muscles. The oxygen clears the lactate from our muscles. So if there is an adequate amount of oxygen, there won't be an accumulation of this lactic acid. This is *aerobic* muscle contraction or muscle contraction in the presence of oxygen. If exercise is rapid or vigorous, the exercising muscle produces lactate faster than oxygen can be supplied to the muscle, lactate accumulates and *oxygen debt* is created in the muscle. The muscle may feel tired or tight. This is due to the accumulation of lactate in the exercising muscle. Continued exercise of the muscle in this state is what is meant by *anaerobic* exercise, exercising the muscle in the absence of oxygen. If the muscle continues to be exercised, more and more lactate accumulates and the oxygen debt and muscle fatigue increase. This kind or exercise, anaerobic exercise, stimulates muscle growth. These physiologic events are used in strength training.

"Then there's the recovery phase of the muscle. Resting the muscle decreases the rate of lactate formation. Deep breathing, bringing more oxygen to the muscle, helps to clear the lactate and decrease the fatigue. That's the payback of the *oxygen debt*.

"Thank your Maker for this. Because of this fantastic mechanism, our muscles are able to contract and perform work in the absence of sufficient oxygen, unlike the motor engines we've invented. Generally, the maximum amount of oxygen that can be exchanged is about four liters a minute. But an athlete who sprints a hundred yards in ten seconds may use six liters of oxygen in the process. After the sprint, the athlete pants and breathes deeply, repaying the oxygen debt over the next several minutes.

"Theoretically, if oxygen is brought to the exercising muscles and clears the lactate at the same rate that the muscle produces it, no lactate is accumulated and there is no oxygen debt. This is the *pay as you go* mechanism. This is *aerobic* exercise, exercise with oxygen. Carefully paced exercises that use the larger muscles of the body like the leg muscles are aerobic, or cardiopulmonary, exercises. Good examples are treadmill exercising, brisk walking, jogging, cycling, and stair stepping among many others. But if aerobic exercises are performed too fast or too long, an anaerobic phase will be entered. Lactate accumulation, oxygen debt, and muscle fatigue will then develop."

"How can we tell if that's happening? If I'm doing an aerobic exercise like brisk walking for a cardiopulmonary workout—how can I tell that I'm entering an anaerobic phase of exercise? That's not what I want to do, is it?" asked Miriam.

"You're right," replied Zinney. "If you're doing an aerobic exercise purely for a cardiopulmonary workout, there's no point in entering into an anaerobic phase. It's counter-productive. While there's no foolproof way of telling when this is happening, a simple rule of thumb is that you should have sufficient breath to carry on a normal conversation while exercising. If you can't talk to someone in a normal conversational manner, then chances are, you are entering an anaerobic phase of exercise. You should slow down; and if that doesn't work, you should stop. When you're able to resume that conversation, you might resume the exercise at a slower pace."

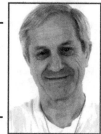

Sam asked, "What kind of exercise burns more calories—aerobic exercise or anaerobic exercise?"

"During exercise you can definitely burn more calories with aerobic exercise than with anaerobic exercise," said Zinney. "You can probably burn more calories in a thirty minute cardiopulmonary workout than you can in an hour or more of strength training.

"But that's not the end of the story. Remember what we've talked about in this regard. Muscles burn calories at rest and larger muscles burn even more calories at rest. By increasing your strength and the muscle mass of your body through strength training, you will actually burn more calories, even at rest. Your metabolic rate will increase. You will be burning more calories all day long."

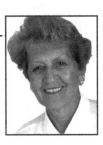

"But if I exercise my legs and my arms, I don't want them to get bigger—I want them to get smaller," said Miriam.

"We talked about this before. You don't have to worry about getting bigger," Zinney responded. "It's not going to happen through strength training unless that's your goal. Studies done on women have repeatedly shown that increasing the muscle mass of thighs by strength training did not increase the actual size of the thighs. They either got smaller or stayed the same size but were better toned—more firm. As the muscle mass increased, the fat mass decreased. Some people are afraid to get into strength training because they genuinely harbor the misconception that they will get to look like a body-builder with big bulging muscles. Building big muscles takes a lot more gym time than what we're talking about. Bodybuilders commonly spend three to six hours a day in the gym five to six days a week. I recommend a strength-training program that takes about thirty minutes two to four times a week. There's a big difference!

"There's a little rap ditty that sums it all up. It goes like this:

> On a pound of fat, let me make
> my case,
> a pound of muscle takes
> less space.
> A pound of muscle, you soon
> will learn,
> hastens the pace of the fat
> you burn.
> So listen up, cat, and hear
> my chat.
> A pound of muscle is where
> it's at.
> A pound of fat is a pound
> of fat,
>
> A pound of fat is only that.

"Well now, let me continue because there's another point I'd like to make about some of the popular aerobic exercises. Jogging and running are great cardiopulmonary exercises, but they're considered high impact exercise and might be responsible for causing joint damage. While there is some merit to these concerns, there's also some value to impact. Exercise associated with impact helps to stimulate those wonderful little osteoblasts—those cells in our bones that produce healthy bone. We already know that strength-training exercises do this dramatically, they increase bone density. But we're not so sure about low impact exercise.

"Low impact exercises like swimming, walking, cycling, and stair stepping are excellent in terms of a cardiopulmonary workout and in terms of reducing joint stress. But because they are of low impact, they may have a lesser effect in preventing osteoporosis. Despite this, walking is in fact a weight bearing exercise; and brisk walks at frequent intervals can actually have a positive effect on bone density. One study, in post-menopausal women, showed that brisk walking for four hours a week reduced hip fractures by 41 percent. For those of you that can't do this, or who rely on these other low impact exercises as a total workout, you might consider jogging in place for sixty seconds a day. The mild impact you experience by so doing, might better stimulate your 'bone makers', the osteoblasts we talked about a few weeks ago. However, this may not be such a good idea for folks with a back or knee problem. So if that's your situation, check with your doctor. He or she should help you decide what exercises are best for you."

Who should exercise—are there any precautions?

"So am I hearing you say that not everyone should exercise?" said Bertha.

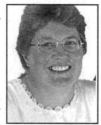

"Well Bertha, that's not what I meant," replied Zinney. "Thomas Jefferson said 'Exercise and recreation…are as necessary as reading. I will rather say more necessary, because health is worth more than learning.' This statement was made about 200 years ago. I'm not sure about the value of making such a comparison. But it emphasizes the enormous respect President Jefferson, who was a scholar of science, had for exercise.

"The Surgeon General reported that failure to exercise, no matter how old you are, might be one of your greatest health hazards, but there are a few exceptions. Some of you may have chronic disorders like heart disease, lung disease, and arthritis. Exercise can benefit you folks as well; but it should be avoided during periods of flare-ups of your illness or what doctors call exacerbations. You can resume your exercise program when you and your doctor believe your flare-up has subsided.

"The important thing for those of us with a chronic condition is stability. Is the condition stable or not? If the condition is stable, then you can start or resume an exercise program. If you have a chronic disease, you have to be educated. You have to know the danger signs that suggest that a flare-up is starting. You and your doctor have to discuss these things so that you understand them. If a symptom develops and you're in doubt as to its importance, check with your doctor. He or she may want you to come in for a checkup before you start or resume your exercise program.

Exercise intensity

"Mild to moderate exercise can benefit almost anyone and more vigorous exercise will benefit most of us even more. Some studies show that people who indulge in mild to moderate activity seem to age as well as those who indulge in more vigorous exercise. These are observational studies that looked at populations who were involved in walking clubs, gardening clubs, and similar endeavors—wonderful ideas. But you are an individual, each and every one of you. As such, the better condition you are in, the better off you will be. Of course fitness can be carried to an extreme. I'm talking about fitness for health not fitness for fitness. The training program of a professional boxer is an example of fitness for fitness. A boxer training for a championship fight would want to be in better condition than his opponent in the last round of the fight. While we appreciate the merits of his endeavor, there's no evidence that his extreme level of fitness provides him with any additional health benefit."

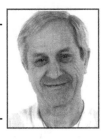

"But, Dr. Zinney, what is vigorous exercise and what's mild?" asked Sam.

"Another good question," Zinney responded. "Generally speaking, exercise that makes you sweat a lot or makes you short of breath is vigorous exercise. Exercise that produces a mild sweat or leaves you slightly winded is moderate exercise. And exercise that does neither is mild exercise. Now understand that mild exercise for one person may be vigorous exercise for another. Also remember, some of us tend to sweat much more easily than others. So these guidelines have to be individualized and learned with experience.

"It's important to start slowly, to start gradually, and to avoid hurting yourself by over-activity. Any good exercise program is likely to be associated with some mild muscular discomfort, but rushing into vigorous exercise can cause injury and pain. This can put you on the sidelines and cause you to lose the gain you've achieved. It can also create a negative psychological feedback that will cause you to avoid exercise. So let's approach it slowly and let's gradually build on the gain we achieve. A little later, we'll explain how to do this with each type of exercise.

"There are some people in whom strength training could be hazardous; and there are others who should avoid any type of vigorous exertion. These are individuals with conditions such as, uncontrolled high blood pressure, certain uncontrolled heart arrythmias, damaged heart valves, aortic aneurysms, unstable angina, recent or untreated congestive heart failure (CHF), and a variety of other chronic conditions during flare-up. For example, if you have rheumatoid arthritis and develop a red-hot inflamed joint, you shouldn't exercise until the acute inflammation is controlled."

"I don't understand what an aortic aneurysm is," said Sheila.

"The aorta is the main artery going out from the heart. It travels down the chest, through the diaphragm, and into the abdomen, giving off branches that supply blood to all parts of the body. Some people are afflicted with a weakening in the wall of this blood vessel so that there is a ballooning out or a bubble formation. In this circumstance, exertion could encourage it to rupture or break and that could be a fatal event [fig. 9A]. Albert Einstein succumbed to a ruptured abdominal aortic aneurysm.

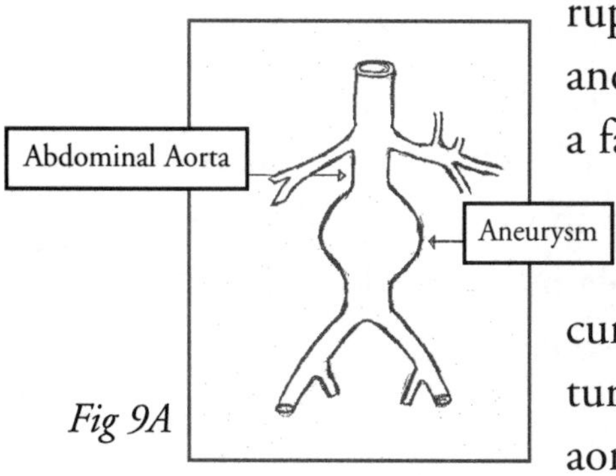

Abdominal Aorta

Aneurysm

Fig 9A

However, if someone had a very small aneurysm or has one surgically repaired, his doctor might prescribe certain exercises that would be ok to do.

Regarding heart valve damage, the heart has four valves, as shown in this slide [fig. 9B]. Certain diseases like rheumatic fever can damage these valves. Sometimes the damage is of such a magnitude that it interferes with the flow of blood into or out of the heart. This can vary with the severity of the damage. If you have such a condition, you should consult your physician regarding your exercise program.

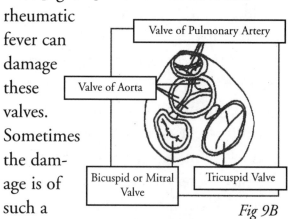

Valve of Pulmonary Artery

Valve of Aorta

Bicuspid or Mitral Valve

Tricuspid Valve

Fig 9B

"The same can be said about coronary artery disease. As you know, coronary diesease can be associated with angina pectoris. This usually causes chest pain on exertion. In mild cases, mild exercise often improves exertional tolerance. But if the angina recurs more frequently, more severely, or with less exertion than previously experienced, it should be checked. As I'm sure you can all appreciate, this is a very serious condition that can lead to a heart attack and can result in fatality. So much can be done today for people with this condition in the form of medication, angioplasty, coronary stent placement, bypass surgery, and the like that it's almost criminal to avoid seeking proper medical care.

"Congestive heart failure (CHF) deserves special consideration particularly because it is so often the cause for hospitalization in older adults. In this condition the heart muscle's pump action is weakened. The volume of blood it pumps out with each beat is decreased. This can result in a back up of fluid in the lungs and other parts of the body like the ankles and legs—a condition called edema. People with this condition can have marked muscle wasting. The weakness can be so marked that they are unable to perform everyday tasks. Resistance training can dramatically improve muscle strength and functionality in these people; and endurance exercises like brisk walking or cycling exercises can improve heart and lung function. But you still need to avoid exercise during flare-ups, or exacerbations. If someone with CHF develops chest discomfort, shortness of breath, or a fluttering in the chest, they should check with their physician.

"Many chronic problems are characterized by alternating periods of exacerbation and remission, when the dis-ease gets better and stabilizes, and periods when it worsens. While this is particularly common in congestive heart failure, it is also true of most other chronic conditions. As we said, exercise should only be practiced when the condition is stable—a rule to be adhered to for all chronic conditions. Exercise that would be enormously beneficial to an individual in a stable condition could be very harmful during a flare-up or during a period of instability.

"This is one good reason why you should know all about your disease. And it should go without saying that anyone with a chronic condition should be under the care of a physician on a regular basis anyway."

"Some of what you said is a little frightening," said Leonard. "Maybe I have CHF or another chronic condition and don't know about it."

"You're right, Leonard. It is possible that a person could have something like silent heart disease that they don't know about—because it hasn't produced any symptoms. But, don't cop out before we start. While there are some people who should be checking with their doctor before they significantly increase their exercise, most of us can get on with it. The National Institute of Aging has a list reasons to check with your physician before starting an exercise program. It's shown in this slide [fig. 9C] and there are copies in the back of the room you can take on your way out tonight.

REASONS TO CHECK WITH YOUR DOCTOR BEFORE EXERCISING
(from the National Institute on Aging)

- *any new, undiagnosed symptom*
- *chest pain*
- *irregular, rapid, or fluttery heart beat*
- *severe shortness of breath*
- *significant, ongoing weight loss that hasn't been diagnosed*
- *infections, such as pneumonia, accompanied by fever*
- *fever itself, which can cause dehydration and a rapid heart beat*
- *acute deep-vein thrombosis (blood clot)*
- *a hernia that is causing symptoms*
- *foot or ankle sores that won't heal*
- *joint swelling*
- *persistent pain or a disturbance in walking after you have fallen (You might have a fracture and not know it, and exercise could cause further injury.)*
- *certain eye conditions, such as bleeding in the retina or detached retina (Before you exercise after a cataract or lens implant, or after laser treatment or other eye surgery, check with your physician.)*

Fig 9C

"Aside from these specific conditions, there are some general precautions to follow. If you're at high risk because you're a smoker, or if you're very obese or if you have a family history of heart disease or diabetes—then you should check with your doctor before dramatically increasing your exertion. So if you're going to do *vigorous* exercise instead of mild or moderate exercise *and* if you're a male over forty or a female over fifty, you should have a medical checkup.

"I think it's a good idea because anyone who *can* do vigorous exercise, *should* do vigorous exercise. And for those of us that can't indulge in vigorous exercise, the vast majority of us should be involved in regular moderate to mild exercise. You know, the second mouse gets the cheese and now it's our chance.

Other precautions

"There are some additional precautions you need to know about. I don't think you should exercise for two hours after a meal. During this time your digestive system is hard at work. Your body knows this and has directed your blood flow towards your digestive tract. Exercise would redirect your blood flow to your muscles and away from your digestive tract—not a good thing. So if you've eaten a hearty meal, rest for at least two hours before starting to exercise.

"Also, some of you have asked me whether you should exercise when you have a cold. The rule of thumb that some have recommended has been the rule of *above the chin or below the chin*. If you have a stuffy nose and a mild sore throat, it's ok to exercise. If you have fever, muscle aches, cough, or shortness of breath—don't exercise. However, some studies have shown that vigorous physical activity can help stimulate the multiplication of viruses. So if you're feeling lousy, I recommend that you take it easy and rest until you're feeling better regardless of whether it's above the chin or below the chin. When you do resume exercise, do it gradually. Start with half the amount of your regular routine for half the amount of time and gradually progress to your full routine."

Where to exercise

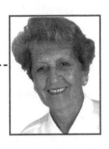

"Where do we do the exercise? Can we do it at home or do we have to join a health club or something?" asked Miriam.

"Excellent question, Miriam. You don't have to join a gym or a health club. Almost all the benefits of exercise can be achieved at home; and you don't need a lot of fancy equipment. However, I know many folks who actually have a gym at home. Keiser, Cybex, Bowflex, and many others manufacturers make excellent equip-

ment that can be used at home. Stretching exercises, balance exercises, endurance exercises, and even strength training can all be done at home. We'll teach you how. I will explain, with the use of diagrams and demonstrations, how to do all of the different kinds of exercise without joining a health club. For many of these exercises, like walking or jogging, all you need is a proper pair of shoes. And if you do it correctly and stay with it—that's great. The problem is that many of us, if not most of us, won't do it at home. We won't do it right; we won't do it regularly; we won't do it enough; or we'll get bored and not do it at all.

"Now I know, that many exercise facilities are noisy and intimidating—with slim girls in leotards and big studs in tank shirts all strutting their fabulous figures and bulging muscles. But many health facilities have special programs for mature adults and seniors. There are some facilities that are dedicated to mature adults, people over the age of forty. There are others that have special hours or sessions and special programs for mature adults.

"In this kind of a program, you can get some individual instruction on what exercises might benefit you as an individual. In other words, we can learn what our individual weaknesses are and how we can best address them with exercise. We can learn the proper form and the best sequence of doing the different exercises. We can have our progress monitored more accurately. If we're making mistakes in our exercise program, they can be identified and corrected more quickly. This can be of importance in preventing injury and improving results.

Group exercise

"Most importantly, at this facility and those with similar programs, we can do it together. We can encourage each other. Each of us can help to motivate each other. We can take pride in our collective progress. We can enjoy each other's company on a regular basis. We'll become a group that can inspire others to form similar groups. This is a fabulous way to make new friends. Jogging clubs, gardening clubs, and neighborhood walking clubs are good examples of this. These clubs combine healthy activity with social interaction.

"If you can be involved in any of these activities, that's great but they're not mutually exclusive to the kind of program we're discussing. The merit of walking clubs is that they encourage exercise and togetherness; but, on the flip side, they don't differentiate the exercise needs of the individual. While walking is a great exercise, if you *can*

do a lot more, you *should* do a lot more. The valuable point here is that people who play together may stay with it together.

"I know clubs may not be everyone's cup of tea. Many people enjoy exercising with more privacy and that's ok too—if you'll do it. For most of you who feel this way, I still think you'd be better served to start a program at a facility like this for eight to sixteen weeks to get initiated and to learn how to do it right. Then if you choose to do all or some of your workouts at home, you'll be better trained, less prone to injury, more disciplined, and more likely to stick with it."

Personal trainers

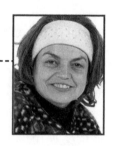

"It sounds to me as if some of us would be better off with a personal trainer. What do you think of that idea?" asked Sheila.

"For some, it's an excellent idea; but it's also more expensive. In selecting a personal trainer, you want to know a lot about their qualifications and experience because almost anyone can call himself or herself a personal trainer. For example, some personal trainers are overzealous in regard to performing exercises through a full range of motion. While range of motion is important, older adults may have significant limitations. Licensed Physical Therapists usually make very good senior fitness trainers because of their experience in dealing with disability and muscle weakness. The level of experience a prospective trainer has had with mature or older adults is important.

"It could help to observe your prospective trainer working with a client. Note how attentive the trainer is to the client's activity. A knowledgeable and attentive personal trainer can be very motivational and have a very positive effect on your progress.

"A good personal trainer may know such things as the effects that certain medications might have on heart rate and blood pressure. In this regard, there are some excellent courses of instruction in adult and senior fitness training that are university affiliated or sponsored by The American College of Sports Medicine. Some fitness organizations and clubs also sponsor excellent programs. But be aware, that some fitness clubs certify trainers after as little as forty-eight hours of instruction. So it's really important that you be diligent in your inquiry as to a prospective trainer's qualifications."

Frequency of exercise

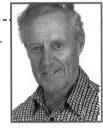

"How often should we exercise—two or three times a week or what?" asked Craig. "I heard that you only have to do cardiopulmonary exercises for twenty or thirty minutes three times a week."

"That seems to be true from a cardiopulmonary standpoint. The frequency and type of exercise is going to vary from one individual to another. Let me give you some general guidelines. You should do stretching exercises every day, and strength, balance, and endurance training two or three days a week. Your individual level of fitness will be an important determinant. Some of us will exercise two or three times a week, combining strength and endurance training. Others will want to workout seven days a week. For example, you might do strength and balance training on Mondays, Wednesdays, and Fridays; and do endurance training on Tuesdays, Thursdays, and Saturdays. On Sundays you would only do stretching—a daily exercise. A seven-day program may sound grueling to some of you because you're not doing it. But believe me—you'll feel so much better you won't know yourself. You'll love it.

"Strength training can be more effectively and more safely done two or three times a week with supervision; and more often than not, with the use of specific resistance machines.

"In this way, a safe range of motion and the proper form can be individually established and imprinted on your mind. Moreover, strength training can be adjusted to encompass a cardiopulmonary workout. Some people can achieve an excellent level of fitness this way and only workout three days a week. We'll get into all this next week.

"So bring your sweat suits and let's get it on! We're gonna have a ton of fun! I look forward to seeing all of you—same station in one week. For those of you that are interested, Joe and his crew will give a tour of the place before you leave."

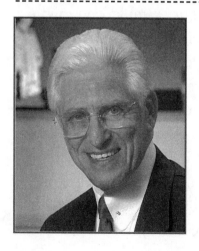

10

Prevent contractures,
Prevent that sprain,
Prevent those fractures,
And hold the gain.

Stretching

It was 10 A.M. and people were assembling in the aerobics room at the fitness center. Zinney couldn't help commenting to Ms. Worthington on the potpourri of attire. Some came in ragged shorts and others in designer sweats and new Adidas cross-trainers. If it wasn't April, you might have thought it was Mardi Gras time.

An obese man, who seemed slightly short of breath, said, "This should be very interesting. The only exercise I've gotten in the last twenty years has been the three S's. You know, Sex, Strenuous coughing and Struggling with a hard bowel movement."

Zinney began, "Well, folks, welcome to the starting line. Here we are in the aerobics room; but we're not here to do aerobics today, we're here to learn stretching exercises. I want us to learn these before we begin our strength-training program. Stretching may not burn many calories or increase strength or endurance, but believe me, stretching exercises are very important to you and to your exercise program. And they only take about five minutes.

"Some recent studies suggest that stretching isn't as important as we thought. That doesn't make any sense to me. As we get older we get stiffer. Our flexibility decreases. Our range of motion decreases. When we exceed our more limited range of motion, we tear or strain muscle and ligament fibers. This causes injury and pain. As we will see later, these injuries can interrupt our exercise program or put us on the sidelines. And the injury can be quite serious.

"Some people believe stretching should be done after a workout; and others believe it should precede the workout. Both are correct. Stretching improves flexibility; it prevents tightening of muscles and freezing of joints. As we age, muscles and tendons tend to tighten and ligaments tend to undergo increasing fibrosis. They may become less elastic and even calcify. This process, together with arthritic changes in the joints, makes us less flexible and more prone to injury. We pull something in our backs when we bend over or in our shoulders when we lift something. Even worse, we don't avoid an oncoming car when we're driving because we don't look in both directions as well as we should. When we twist an ankle or fall, we have a greater tendency to tear ligaments or develop a fracture—all because of a lack of flexibility."

"I don't understand," said Craig. "First of all, what's the difference between tendons and ligaments? And how does this tightening increase fractures?"

"Well, look at this slide [fig. 10A]. A tendon is that part of the muscle that attaches to the bone.

"When the muscle contracts it moves the bone. This picture shows the biceps muscle, you know, that big muscle in the front of your upper arm. The tendon attaches to the forearm and, when it contracts and shortens, it bends the arm.

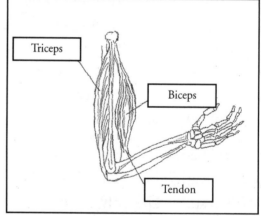

Fig 10A

"Ligaments, on the other hand, are firm fibrous structures that support the various joints in our body, as shown in this slide [fig. 10B].

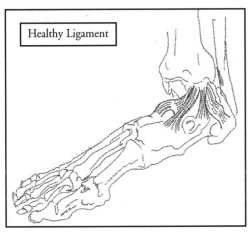

Fig 10B

"In the next diagram [fig. 10C], you see a joint with sclerotic or hardened ligaments undergoing flexion.

"As you can see, the joint with the sclerotic ligament, being less elastic,

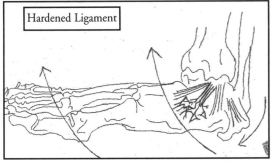

Fig 10C

has a tendency to tear some of its fibers. It even tore a piece of bone with it. It caused a fracture!

"So a lack of flexibility increases your chances of sprains, torn ligaments, and muscle strains. It decreases your range of motion, how far you can move your arms, legs, neck, or any part of your body in different directions. A decreased range of motion during exercise decreases the benefit of the actual exercise, simply because

you're moving your limbs a shorter distance during each exercise. It also increases the risk of injury during exercise. So you can see why I believe that if you stretch for life, you just might stretch your life.

The principles of stretching

"Before getting into the specifics of each exercise, there are some important concepts I want to share with you that apply to all stretching exercises. Mild stretching before a workout is a good idea; but you should warm up first by swinging your arms, walking a little, and/or jogging in place for a minute or two. Stretching cold muscles can sometimes result in injury. After a workout, your muscles are pumped and tight; so it's particularly important to do stretching at the end of each exercise session.

"But there are even more important things to remember. Stretching is not a competitive sport. If the guy next to you can touch his toes and you can't, that's not important. Beating him is not your goal. Your goal is to improve your own flexibility, or even more importantly, to prevent it from decreasing as you age. Also, stretching exercises should not be painful. They should make you feel good and more limber.

161

"If you're experiencing pain while stretching, then you're stretching too much or too far. Each movement should be slow and deliberate, not jerky. And each stretch should be maintained for fifteen to thirty seconds and then repeated two to four more times. Many people rush through their stretching maneuvers. Don't be impatient. Stretch slowly. It will make you feel great. Also, do not lock your joints while doing a movement; but allow them to bend slightly.

"If a particular movement produces pain, then back off a little and stretch to a point short of causing pain. Very gradually increase your stretch with each movement over a period of weeks. When you've reached your limit, you've achieved your goal, a new and flexible you. You should strive to maintain this new and wonderful level of flexibility by stretching at least three times a week, preferably every day.

"If you've had surgery on your hip, knee, or back, or any other kind of major orthopedic surgery, your doctor might not want you to do certain types of stretching exercises. So check with your physician first. For example, if you've had a hip replacement, I wouldn't want you to cross your legs and I wouldn't want you to bend your hips more than ninety degrees.

Floor exercises (getting up and down)

"Since many stretching exercises are done on the floor, special care has to be taken if you've had hip replacement surgery or if you have a bad back. Some people are fearful about lying on the floor because they may have difficulty in getting back up. If any of you have this concern, it's best for you to use a buddy system for floor exercises. Have someone assist you in getting down and up.

"In the absence of a buddy, you can get into and back up from a lying position by a series of movements that Georgina, one of our fitness trainers, will demonstrate. First, put your hands on the seat of a sturdy chair [fig. 10D].

"Then lower yourself down on one knee and follow by bringing the other knee down [fig. 10E].

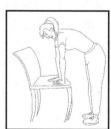

Fig 10D

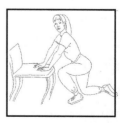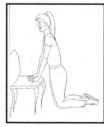

Fig 10E

"Put one hand on the floor and keep one hand on the seat of the chair as you lower yourself onto your hip (fig. 10F).

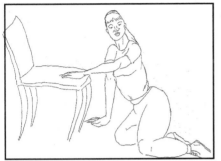

Fig 10F

"Now your weight is on your hip and you are lying on your side. From here, you can roll over onto your back [fig. 10G].

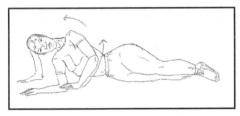

Fig 10G

"To get up, you can roll back onto your side and place your hands on the floor at about the level of your upper chest [fig. 10H].

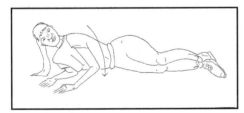

Fig 10H

"Then push your shoulders off the floor and, while leaning on your hands for support, shift your weight in the direction of your knees so that you are on all fours.

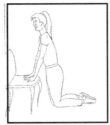
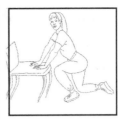

Fig 10I

"Lean your hands on the seat of the chair and lift one of your legs so that your foot is flat on the floor [fig. 10I].

"Now rise up using your legs and hands. That having been said, let's get on with some of the specifics. We'll start with the upper body.

Neck exercises

"When doing neck-stretching exercises, it's a good idea to be seated comfortably in a straight back chair. It's really important to do these slowly because sudden changes in the position of the head can cause dizziness, particularly in people who have inner ear problems. Be sure to avoid a bouncing motion. Also, if you've had any neck or back problems, be sure your doctor thinks these exercises are ok for you.

"All of you take a seat in one of the chairs facing the front of the room. The two chairs in the front that are facing you are for Sheila and Sam. They're going to be our demonstration subjects for these exercises. I'll demonstrate the exercises on them; and Georgina and Joe will wander among you to supervise your performance as all of us do the movements together.

"Sheila! Sam! Come on up here and have a seat."

Sheila eagerly accepted the offer of celebrity but Sam was surprisingly shy. He said, "Thanks, Doc, but I'm not sure. Why don't you pick someone else?"

"Sam, you're our man for this. You are the man!" said Zinney as he encouraged Sam to take a demonstration seat.

"To stretch the back of your neck, slowly bend your head forward trying to put your chin on your chest until you feel a pleasant stretching sensation in the back of your neck [fig. 10J]. Hold this position for fifteen seconds, then slowly return to the straight up position.

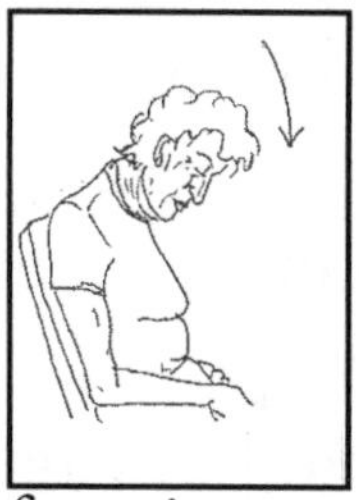

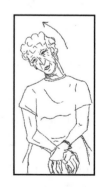

Fig 10J

"Let's repeat it three or four times. Straighten up slowly between each movement, no jerky movements. Very good, folks.

"For the front of your neck, slowly bend your head back to look up at the ceiling until you feel a pleasant stretching sensation in the front of your neck [fig. 10K]. Do this exercise in a chair with a supportive straight back to avoid leaning backwards. Hold this position for ten to fifteen

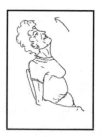

Fig 10K

seconds and return to the resting position slowly. Repeat the movement three to five times. Don't rush. Each time you are at your full stretch, open and close your mouth slowly to count the seconds. Hum a M-M-M each time you close your mouth for a second. This will help to stretch the tissues in the front of your neck. Come on let's hear that M-M-M all together. Good! Great going, Sam and Sheila. Now, guys and gals, doesn't that feel great? You bet it does! All right, let's repeat this two more times.

"Now for the sides of your neck. Look straight ahead and tilt your head towards one shoulder and then towards the other shoulder [fig. 10L].

"As always, do it slowly and hold the stretch for ten to twenty seconds; and repeat the movement three to five times. It's a good idea to do this movement in front of a mirror so you can avoid raising or shrugging your shoulder towards your head. The object is not

Fig 10L

to touch the side of your head with your shoulder, but simply to stretch both sides of your neck. Remember, no jerking motions. Very good! Hey, you're doing real good, Sam. You too, Sheila, keep it up.

"Okay, let's do some neck rotation exercises. Now you can do these exercises lying on the floor with a firm pillow or a book under your head [fig. 10M], or you can do them in the sitting position.

"Since we're all sitting already, that's how we'll do them. Look straight ahead, keeping the head in a level position, not looking down or up. Start by turning your head first to the left side as far as it will go, just to a level of mild discomfort and hold it there for fifteen seconds. That's good, very good. Now, go back to the forward viewing position then turn your head very slowly to the right and hold it there for fifteen seconds. Now back again to the forward viewing position. Let's repeat this two more times."

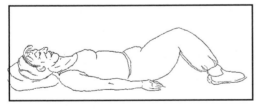

Fig 10M

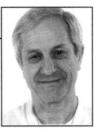

"That's the sound of your old rusty hinges," replied Zinney. "Snapping or popping sounds are common in stretching exercises but they're not dangerous. However, if you have a medical history of neck problems, you should check with your doctor before doing these exercises. The important thing to remember is not to stretch to the point of causing pain. Do it slowly and deliberately.

Arms and shoulders

"Now we're going to stretch our arms and our shoulders. For these exercises, I want Craig and Miriam to come up here. It's probably better for all of you folks to be standing up while we're trying this one. We're going to use a towel to stretch the muscles and the ligaments of our upper arms, shoulders, and elbows. Hold the towel with your right hand and drape it over your back [fig. 10N]. Bend your elbow so that the towel falls down your back and then grasp the towel with your left hand behind your back. Gradually

165

grasp it higher and higher up the towel with your left hand. This stretches your triceps, shoulders, and elbows. Hold this position for 10 to 20 seconds and then reverse your hands. Just stretch until it's comfortable or a little bit uncomfortable, but no pain, no jerky motions. Hold the stretch for 10 to 20 seconds.

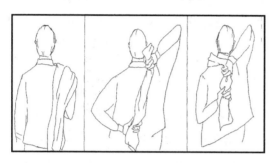

Fig 10N

"Now reverse your hands so that your left hand is on top and put your right hand behind your back to grasp the lower end of the towel. Again, gradually inch your right hand closer and closer to your left until you feel a mild stretching sensation in your shoulders, upper arms, and elbows.

"Repeat this two more times and hold that stretch for 10 to 20 seconds. See how much more limber you feel.

"Next, lie down on the mat in front of your chair using the technique we described earlier for getting into the lying position. There's a pillow for each of you. Lie on the floor with your head straight and knees slightly bent.

"Bend your arms at the elbow with your hands facing straight up [fig. 10O]. Slowly drop your hands down with your elbows still bent at a right angle so that your fingers are pointing towards your toes.

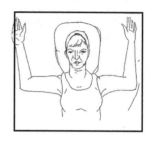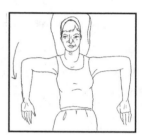

Fig 10O

"Then, raise your hands upward very slowly with your elbows still at right angles so that your fingers are pointing in the direction of your head again. As soon as you feel a stretch or slight discomfort, that's where you stop. Don't try to stretch too far.

"Do it slowly and maintain each position for 10 to 20 seconds. Now slowly let your arms roll forward pointing your fingers down toward your feet again. Stop as soon as you feel a mild stretch or discomfort—no pain or jerking motions. Hold each position for 10 to 30 seconds. Remember to keep your shoulders and elbows on the floor and your arms bent at ninety degrees. Repeat the movements three to five times.

Wrist and hands

"Ok. Let's all get up and sit in our chairs. We're going to do some stretching of the wrists and hands. Put your hands together in front of your chest as if you were praying [fig. 10P].

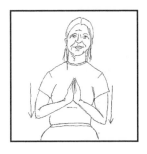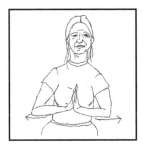

Fig 10P

"Keep the heels of your hands and the fingertips together. Slowly raise your elbows while keeping your hands together. You'll feel a slight stretching sensation in your wrists and fingers. Hold it for 10 to 30 seconds.

"Now relax and repeat this movement two or three more times holding the stretch position for fifteen to twenty seconds each time.

Outer thighs and hips

"Next, we're going to get back on the floor to stretch the muscles of our thighs and our hips. If any of you have had hip surgery, don't do this exercise until your physician approves it. The starting position is on our backs with a pillow under our heads,

our shoulders flat, and our knees bent. We have to keep our feet flat on the floor and our knees together [fig. 10Q].

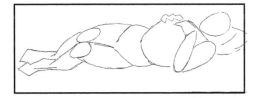

Fig 10Q

"Let's gently rotate our knees, first to the right side as far as possible [fig. 10R], but without any pain—just until we feel a mild stretch. Hold this position for about fifteen seconds, and go back to the starting position. Then rotate your knees to the left side just until we feel a mild stretch. Hold that stretch for fifteen seconds.

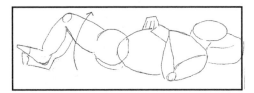

Fig 10R

"Repeat the movement two or three more times to each side and hold the stretch for fifteen to twenty seconds each time.

Quadriceps

"Now, let's stretch our quadriceps. Those are the muscles in the front

167

of our thighs. Start by rolling on your side. Again, if you've had hip surgery please check with your physician before doing this exercise. Let's roll on the left side, bend our right knee, and hold onto our foot with our right hand. If you can't reach your foot, loop a towel over the top of your right foot and grasp the towel with your right hand [fig. 10S].

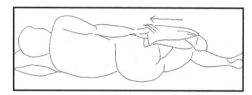

Fig 10S

"Then, gently pull on the towel until you feel a mild stretching sensation in the front of your right thigh and in your knee.

"Hold the stretch for fifteen to twenty seconds, then roll onto your right side and repeat the movement. Let's do this two or three times on each side and hold the stretch for fifteen to twenty seconds each time. This can also be effective in stretching the front of your ankle. You folks are doing just great. Let's keep going!

Inner thighs

"Now let's roll on our backs and stretch the muscles on the inner aspect of our thighs. But, again, if you've had hip surgery, check with your doctor

before you do this exercise. The starting position for this movement is lying flat on our backs. Bend your right knee upwards toward your head then slowly lower it towards the floor in a sideways direction keeping your back and pelvis flat on the floor [fig. 10T].

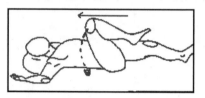

Fig 10T

"Now do this until you feel a mild stretch and hold it for about fifteen seconds. Then return to the starting position by bringing your knee slowly back into place. Repeat this again with each leg two or three times and hold the stretch for fifteen seconds each time. Keep your shoulders flat and keep your hips and pelvis flat on the floor. Excellent. You're all doing great.

Back of the thighs

"As you can see, we brought in a bunch of benches. This is for doing a hamstring stretch. Those are the muscles in the back of your thigh. Now once again, if you've had hip replacement surgery or any major hip surgery, you have to check with your physician before doing these exercises. Okay, now Craig and Miriam, each of you take one of these benches and sit sideways on the bench. All of you follow suit. Everyone sit sideways on the bench and put one leg stretched out on the bench [fig. 10U].

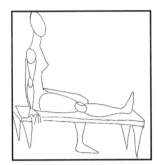

Fig 10U

"That's it, straight out on the bench. The other leg is off the bench with your foot flat on the floor. Don't lock that leg on the bench. It doesn't have to be absolutely straight if it causes you too much discomfort.

"Gradually lean forward very slowly from the hips. Do not bend at the waist. When you feel that stretching in the back of your leg, hold it there for fifteen seconds. Don't cause yourself any pain. Stop bending forward when you feel that mild stretching sensation. Hold it for around fifteen seconds. That's very good. Now just relax and let your leg on the bench bend a little bit. Let's repeat this movement two or three more times with each leg and hold the stretch for about fifteen seconds.

"But remember the important elements of this movement are as follows: the foot that's on the floor

should be kept flat on the floor and your shoulders should be kept straight throughout the movement.

"Gradually—very gradually bend forward at the hips, not at the waist until you feel that mild stretching sensation in the back of your leg. Hold it for fifteen seconds. Do it slowly, no jerking motions. [fig. 10V].

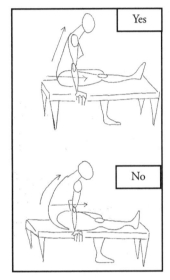

Fig 10V

"For those of you who don't have a bench at home, there is an alternative method of doing a hamstring stretch using a straight-back chair. Let me show you. Come on, Craig. Stand behind the chair keeping your legs straight. Hold the back of the chair with both hands and bend forward from the hips, not your waist [fig. 10W]. You have to keep your back and your shoulders straight throughout the entire maneuver, until your upper body is parallel to the floor.

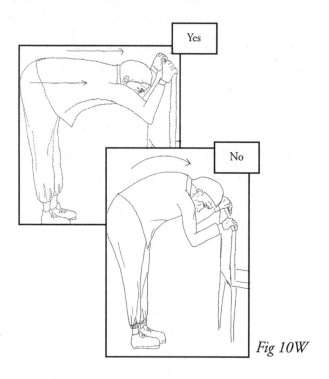

Yes

No

Fig 10W

"Again, hold this position for fifteen seconds and repeat the movement three to five times. Do it slowly, without any jerking; and don't, don't hump your back. Very good, Craig.

"Well, Joe, how are the folks you're supervising doing over there?"

"Are you kidding?! These people will be ready for the Olympics in a few weeks. They're doing wonderfully!"

Calf muscles

Zinney continued, "To stretch our calves, stand up and put your hands against the wall, keeping your arms straight. Step back with one leg about 1 to 2 feet with both knees slightly bent. Keep your back foot flat on the floor.

"Gradually straighten your back knee, but keep your front knee slightly bent [fig. 10X]. You should feel a pleasant stretch in the back of your calf. Just hold that position for about fifteen seconds. Do it with the other leg. Hold it again for fifteen seconds. Repeat this movement with each leg two or three more times.

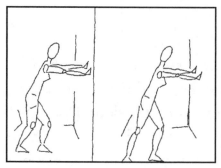

Fig 10X

Back stretching movements

"Next, we're going to stretch the creaky ligaments and muscles of our tired old backs. Many of us get up each morning with a sore back.

"Often this is the result of a bad mattress or a poorly supportive one. A firmer or more supportive mattress could go a long way in solving this problem. Some have even found it beneficial to put a bed board made of 3/4 inch plywood under the mattress; however, others have found it necessary to get a mattress with a greater degree of segmental support.

170

"If chronic low back pain is a problem, it can also help to sleep on your back, not your stomach, with a pillow under your knees. This will help you keep your knees slightly bent and reduce the tension on your low back muscles.

"You can often loosen your stiff and aching back muscles at the side of your bed before actually standing up. Let me demonstrate using this bench as the side of a bed. Sit at the side of your bed with your feet flat on the floor [fig. 10Y].

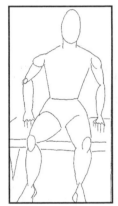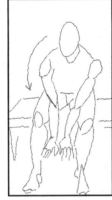

Fig 10Y

"Then gradually bend at the hips, not at the waist, by dropping your shoulders and your arms forward between your knees. Keep the palms of your hands facing the floor and bend forward until you feel a pleasant stretching sensation in your low back. Hold the stretch for ten to fifteen seconds. You don't have to touch the floor with your hands; but as your flexibility improves, you may be able to actually

put the palms of your hands flat on the floor. Do this movement slowly and repeat it two or three times.

"You can do the same kind of low back stretch in a chair. Come on up here, Leonard, and sit in this chair for a demonstration." Leonard quickly sprang to his feet and assumed a seat in the chair facing sideways to the audience. "Leonard, fold your arms in front of your chest and let your shoulders and your head bend forward so that your head drops between your knees [fig. 10Z].

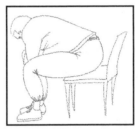

Fig 10Z

"You should feel a mild stretching of your lower back."

"Yeah! I do," Leonard said. "That feels good, Doc."

"Hold the stretch for ten to fifteen seconds. Remember, try to bend mostly at the hips, not the waist. Go back to the starting position and repeat this movement two or three more times.

"Everyone get down on the floor now for some more back exercises. We'll lie on our backs with a pillow under our heads and our knees bent [fig. 10AA]. Keep your shoulders flat and your knees together. Bend your knees up towards your chest and clasp your hands around your knees.

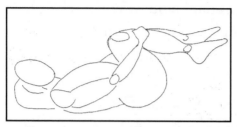

Fig 10AA

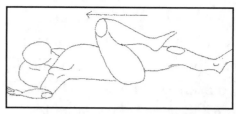

Fig 10BB

"Gently pull your knees towards your chest and hold this stretch for ten to fifteen seconds then return to the starting position.

"Hey! Doesn't that feel great? You betcha it does. Okay, let's repeat the movement two or three more times. Just a couple more movements while we're all still on the floor.

"Let's use the same starting position. Lie flat on your back with your knees bent, shoulders flat, and arms above your head. Move one knee as far as you can towards your chest, and at the same time straighten the other leg [fig. 10BB]. Hold this position for ten seconds and then repeat the movement with the other side. Let's do this two or three more times.

"A lot of people don't realize that one of the most important aspects of maintaining a healthy back is maintaining good abdominal muscle tone. I can't emphasize this enough. Good tone to your abdominal muscles decreases the drag on your low back. We'll get into strengthening the status of our abdominal muscles when we start our strength training.

"However, while we're on our backs there is one exercise I'd like you to try. It's called the 'flat back position.' The starting position is flat on our back, with our knees bent, and our feet flat on the floor. Now, let's try to tighten our abdominal muscles and at the same time tighten our buttocks. This tends to flatten your back against the mat. It requires some concentration and coordination to do this; but once you get it, it's both a good abdominal and a good back exercise. Let's all try it again. Ready and go. Tighten those muscles in your abdomen and your butt. Hold it for five seconds and repeat it several times.

"Well, how do you all feel? Do you feel great—more limber, more stretched? None of you should be in any pain. If you are, you stretched a little too far and you'll have to be more careful next time...

"Ok! We're going to go across the hall where we're going to learn about resistance training. It's time to start our engines and build our strength. So, everybody up – rise and shine. And let's go right across the hall."

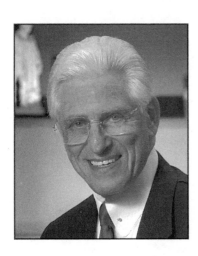

11

More muscle will build
From the sweat you have spilled.
So please try to continue
To bring forth what's in you.

Strength Training

"Look at this room, will you," said Miriam. "It's got mirrors all over the place."

"Yeah, talk about being narcissistic. Some people never get tired of looking at themselves," added Craig.

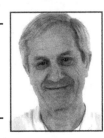

Sam joked, "These machines look like they're made for torture."

"I couldn't help but overhear your fun," said Zinney. "But those machines are not for torture. They're for pleasure. They will pleasure your muscles with a deep massage, a massage that resistance training, and only resistance training, can accomplish. As you contract and stretch each muscle against resistance, every fiber in that muscle can be called into play. And as

the muscle fatigues, it produces the pleasant sensation of internal massage. This releases your endorphins, making you feel great. It makes you feel alive.

The house of mirrors and machines

"You've all heard the comment about resistance training: no pain, no gain. Well, that may be true for bodybuilders and competitive weight lifters; but not for us. It doesn't have to hurt and it shouldn't hurt. Sure, you may have to strain yourself, but you don't have to sprain yourself. Our motto will be 'Strain a little, Gain a lot.' You should feel a pleasant kind of muscle soreness after a workout but no real pain. As your muscle fatigues it will get tight and pumped with blood. You'll feel a soothing warm sensation or a slight burn in the muscle; and then you'll do a little more and rest the muscle. Then, when it's recovered, we may repeat the process and so on. That's how we'll build the strength and the tone of our muscles. And as we've previously said, the really good thing about it is that it's going to happen quickly. All of you are going to be much stronger in just eight weeks.

"The mirrors that you laughed at, Sam, serve a very important practical purpose. By watching yourself do these exercises, you can observe your form. Doing the exercises with proper form and maintaining proper form throughout the exercise is extremely important in getting the maximum benefit from the exercise and avoiding injury. It's true, some us are more vain than others. We may enjoy looking at ourselves more than others. As our physiques improve, all of us might enjoy looking at ourselves more. There's nothing wrong with that. But the real purpose of the mirrors is to help you maintain the proper form for the performance of the various movements we're going to teach you.

"Okay, folks," Zinney continued, "now we're going to start our resistance training program. We're going to make ourselves stronger. We're going to improve our endurance and our balance. And we're going to do this, first, by strengthening our muscles. We're also going to increase the density of our bones and improve our cardiopulmonary function and even our brain function. As you've heard me say many times before, strength training is the single most important kind of exercise and the single most important thing you can do to prevent frailty and maintain your independence. It's the key that will unlock the door to better balance and better cardiopulmonary health. It can increase your muscle mass and reduce your body fat. It can increase your metabolic rate so that you'll burn more calories—even when you're not exercising. Many of you will become as strong or stronger than you were twenty years ago, all during the next eight weeks!"

Craig leaned over and whispered to Sam, "I know that I'm already stronger than I used to be twenty years ago."

"How's that?" asked Sam.

"Well, twenty years ago, when I'd get an erection, I could never bend it. Now I can bend it in every direction," laughed Craig.

Pneumatics, variable resistance, and inertia

"As you look around the room you can see an array of free weights and a wide variety of machines. Some are variable resistance machines and others are pneumatic."

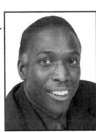

"What do you mean by variable resistance and pneumatic? And why is that important?" asked Leonard.

"To fully appreciate their importance, we should review the concept of inertia. The law of inertia is one of the simple laws of physics. I'll paraphrase it by stating the following: Things at rest tend to stay at rest and things in motion tend to stay in motion. Because of this, it requires more effort or power to start a weight in motion than to keep it moving. You know, it's easier to continue to push a car after it has started rolling than it is to get it moving from a dead stop; and it's also harder to stop it after it's in motion.

"The same is true with moving weight in resistance exercises. It requires more power to get the weight moving from the starting position of the exercise than to keep it moving after you've put it in motion and more effort to stop it on returning to the starting position. Because of this, starting the weight in motion and stopping the weight on the return can cause tearing of some muscle and ligament fibers. This can cause soreness and decrease the effectiveness and enjoyment of your exercise. It may cause a negative psychological feedback that will discourage further exercise.

"The starting point of each exercise with variable resistance machines, such as those made by Nautilus, Cybex, Medex, and others, start with a weight-resistance considerably less than the weight-resistance at the mid point of the exercise. In other words, the machines are engineered so that the resistance gradually increases from the starting point of the exercise to the midpoint of the movement. This is very good because your muscles have less power at the starting point of each exercise and are stronger at the mid-point of the movement. So, you will be able to exercise with more weight at the midpoint of the exercise with a variable resistance apparatus. This can allow you to progress more rapidly, to get stronger in a shorter period of time. Even more importantly, it tends to significantly decrease the effects of inertia and the stress on joints and muscle fibers.

177

"In this regard, pneumatic machines, like those made by the Keiser Company, are very good. They're not associated with inertia. Here, the resistance that you push or pull against is air pressure. And you can increase or decrease the air pressure with conveniently-placed control buttons. These are among my personal favorites. Wherever you exercise after we've completed our course together, try to use exercise machines that decrease the effects of inertia."

Free weights

"What about free weights?" asked John.

"Free weights are wonderful. You can get a great workout with them and build enormous strength. Professional bodybuilders and competitive weightlifters use them extensively. But free weights will subject your joints and muscles to the effects of inertia. Consequently, there is a tendency to swing the weight and cheat on form. So when using free weights, even greater diligence to form is essential. There are some exercises that are actually best performed with free weights. We'll be doing some of them. For starters, however, I'd rather we develop a reasonable level of fitness with resistance machines before we use them too much. Regardless of the type of resistance training you choose—whether it's free weights, weight machines, or whatever—you can get very strong, very toned, very well defined, and even very big if you want to.

Reps and sets

"The jargon of resistance training consists of two terms: reps and sets. The term 'rep' is short for repetition, meaning the performance of an exercise movement from the starting position through the entire range of motion and then back to the starting position. That's what a rep or repetition means. Each repetition or rep consists of a positive and a negative phase. The positive phase of each rep consists of moving against the resistance, or moving the weight from the starting position to the end point of the movement. The negative phase consists of returning the weight-resistance back to the starting position. Both phases of the rep are equally important and should be done slowly, deliberately, and with perfect form. Both phases exercise and strengthen your muscles. And remember this— slow movements, lighter weights, and good form are better than quick movements, heavier resistance, and sloppy form.

"The positive and negative phase of every rep should each be done to the count of four and held at its end point for the count of one. A simple trick that may work for some of you is to use the word 'repetition.' Repetition is a four-syllable word. You can use this word to count your reps and to do each rep to the count of four. For example, count to yourself— RE-PE-TI-TION ONE during the positive phase of the movement and repeat RE-PE-TI-TION ONE during the negative phase. Then count RE-PE-TI-TION TWO for the positive phase of the second rep and RE-PE-TI-TION TWO for the negative phase of the second rep. Then repetition three, four, and so on.

"The number of consecutive reps that you do of any one exercise is called a 'set.' This may vary from as little as three reps to as many as twenty reps in a set. But for our purposes, we'll use eight to fifteen reps in each set. The number of sets for any one exercise will vary from one to five sets, with rest periods between each set that will vary from 45 seconds to 2.5 minutes.

"It's important to approach this gradually. Each of us will progress at a different rate and each of us will have a different level of tolerance in terms of how much we can or even how much we should do. But the important thing is that all of us should do it and all of us will improve. Some of us should only do one set of repetitions for each movement three to four times a week. On the other hand, some of us should only do it twice a week while still others will progress dramatically, doing three or more sets of each exercise every other day. But all of us—every one of us—will gain in strength, vigor, and energy. Even more exciting is that you'll do it in eight weeks. And you'll love it.

"I can't help but notice many of you gawking at the numerous machines in this room. Each one is designed to improve the strength of a specific group of muscles. As you can see, there appears to be no end to the number of contrivances developed for strength training. While you can use all of them later on if you so choose, we're first going to concentrate our efforts on a select few in an effort to establish a substantial degree of fitness.

Principles of resistance training

"The principles of using each one of these machines are the same in terms of reps, sets, and rest periods. You must position yourself correctly, use the proper form and the proper breathing techniques when performing each exercise. We'll show you how to do that.

"First, perform the movement on each machine with no resistance. This will help in establishing the proper form for each movement as well as the proper range of motion for each of us. Having done this, warm up that set of muscles by using a very slight amount of resistance. Do about five repetitions with this minimal resistance. Then, rest approximately two and a half minutes. Next, we will increase the resistance and repeat five repetitions and then rest again. Now we can attempt to see how much resistance you can manage with a one-time effort. For practical purposes, we will call this your maximum effort, also referred to as your 'max' for that exercise. It's very important that you don't hold your breath in performing this maximum movement. You can probably move more weight or more resistance if you were to hold your breath, but that's not the way I want you to do the exercise. I'll explain more about this shortly.

"After determining how much you can lift with your maximum effort, use 75 percent of that weight for your exercises. We'll do the same for each machine or exercise. If your max on one machine or exercise is 100 pounds then we'll do five to eight reps using 75 pounds. If your max on another machine is 80 pounds, then we'll use 60 pounds. If your max on still anoth-er machine is 40 pounds, we'll do five to eight reps using 30 pounds. Each time we do an exercise, we're going to perform five to eight repetitions with perfect form. We're going to perform the positive and negative phase of each rep slowly to a count of four.

"After each set, we rest. We may rest for as little as 45 seconds or for as much as two and half minutes before starting the second set. This will vary from person to person. Some of us will only do one set of each exercise until we get better conditioned, and others will be able to do two or even three sets at each station. We will gradually increase the number of reps to eight and the number of sets to three, while decreasing the rest periods between sets down to 45 or 90 seconds. This should be done gradually over a period of weeks, not days.

"The last rep of the last set should be the most difficult. It should feel as if you can't do one more rep no matter what—you're out of gas. When it doesn't feel that way, when it feels as if you've got more fuel in your tank, it means you've become stronger and it's time to progress to the next step. But do it gradually. Remember today is the first day of the rest of your life. There's no rush.

"The next step consists of increasing the number of reps in each set to ten and then to twelve or more. When you've achieved this and you still have fuel in your tank, you can increase the number of reps in each set to fifteen. Alternatively, you can increase the weight-resistance and start with eight reps in each set again because you're stronger. Isn't that great? It's going to happen to all of you, believe me.

Frequency of training sessions

"Now as we said, for some of you, one set of each exercise two to three times a week will be sufficient, but many of you will want to progress to two or three or more sets. Most of us will work out three or four times a week but some of us will workout almost every day. If you exercise every day, it's important that you avoid exercising the same muscles every day. You might work your upper body on one day and your lower body the next.

"Your muscles become stronger while you're resting, not while you're exercising. All the biochemical reactions that strength training calls into play to make your muscles stronger take about forty-eight hours to produce their effects. So, you want to work different muscles on alternate days. Or as we said earlier, do a complete strength-training workout two or three days a week alternating with endurance training three days a week.

But remember to do stretching exercises every day."

"There are around twenty to thirty different machines here. Which ones are we gonna use?" asked Leonard.

"After a while, you may end up using all of the machines in this room; but first, we're starting with a group of resistance exercises that will produce good fitness in all of our major muscle groups. The following machines are those that will achieve this the best:

- seated bench press—exercises your chest muscles, shoulder muscles, and the triceps muscle in the back of your arm

- seated shoulder or vertical press—exercises your shoulder muscles, upper back muscles, and triceps muscles

- triceps machine—exercises your triceps muscles

- arm curl machine—exercises your biceps and other muscles in the front of your arm

- seated leg press—exercises the muscles in your thigh and calf

- seated leg curl machine—exercises the muscles in the back of your thigh (hamstrings)

- seated leg extension machine—exercises the muscles in the front of your thigh (quadriceps)

- upper back machine—exercises the muscles of your upper back, shoulders, and arms

- upper pull down machine or lat bar—exercises the mid and lower latismus muscle

- abdominal crunch machine—exercises your abdominal muscles

"With the few exceptions that we'll discuss later, the principles of good strength training on all machines are the same. Keep in mind at all times that strength training is not an ego game. It's easy for this to occur.

"If you attempt to increase the resistance too rapidly, you can hurt yourself. Most of us can move more resistance by throwing caution to the wind in terms of not adhering to the proper form for the exercise or by holding our breath. Not only will this increase the likelihood of injury, but also it will cheat you from getting the maximum benefit from the exercise. I can't say it too often, so I'll say it again: good form and good breathing techniques are both essential to good exercise."

Breathing

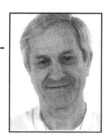

"I would have thought that breathing is a natural thing. Is there something special about it that we should know?" asked Sam.

"Indeed there is," Zinney answered. "There is a natural tendency to hold your breath when doing resistance training. That's the wrong thing to do. Breathing is extremely important and I think we should review a little bit of what happens. There is a flap in the back of your throat that protects the glottis, the opening to your windpipe (trachea), called the epiglottis [fig. 11A].

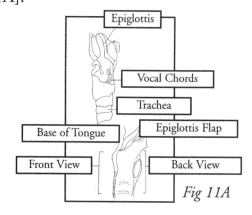

Fig 11A

"This flap, or epiglottis, opens and closes the glottis as you inhale and exhale air. It also prevents food and other unwanted material from getting into your windpipe.

"To hold your breath, the epiglottis, shown in this diagram [fig. 11B], can be closed over the opening to the trachea or the glottis.

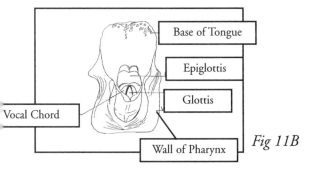

Base of Tongue

Epiglottis

Glottis

Vocal Chord

Wall of Pharynx

Fig 11B

"This is what a lot of you do when you strain to lift something or when you strain to have a hard bowel movement. You take a deep breath and you force an exhalation against a closed glottis.

"When you do this, when you perform this grunting maneuver, you dramatically increase the pressure within your chest and abdomen. This raises your blood pressure and increases the pressure on the organs and blood vessels in your chest. You can do this gently, for example, when you're swimming under water or whenever you hold your breath. But when you do this forcefully, you are compressing your internal organs and producing an adverse effect on your circulatory system.

"When the pressure on the major veins in your chest is increased, it slows the return of blood from the rest of your body to your chest and heart. Since your heart is receiving less blood, it has less blood to pump out with each beat to the very muscles you're exercising. This is the type of straining that even some professional bodybuilders and competitive weightlifters use. But that's not what our training program is about.

"You need to breathe easily throughout the exercise movements. At the beginning of each exercise, we take a deep breath and as we perform the positive movement against resistance, we exhale to the count of four or to the four-syllable word 'repetition.'

"We should complete the exhalation at the same time we complete the positive phase of each rep. And then as we perform the negative phase of each rep by returning to our starting position, we inhale and fill our lungs with air. This sounds very easy; but it's even easier to do it incorrectly. So concentrate on your breathing throughout your entire exercise session; and shortly, it will become second nature to you.

Warm up and cool down

"There are some additional points I want to emphasize. Warming up is one of them and cooling down is another. Do your stretching exercises and warm up the muscles you're going to exercise. You can do this by doing five to eight reps with half or less of the weight-resistance you're going to use for your workout. Take a rest period and then repeat this with a little more weight-resistance. You should do this on each machine. Also, when you've completed your entire workout on all of the machines, you should cool down rather than stop cold. This can usually be accomplished by some brisk walking for a few minutes followed by slower pace walking for a few minutes. Then do your stretching exercises.

Pre-fatigue

"An efficient method of working out is to exercise muscles that are already partially worked out by a prior movement. So, if the seated bench press works out your chest, shoulders, and triceps, and the seated shoulder press works out your shoulders and triceps; it might save time to do them sequentially. You will have partially fatigued some of the same muscles with one exercise and may be able to get an excellent workout on the second machine with a lesser number of reps or sets without sacrificing any benefit.

"Let me take this a bit further. Having pre-fatigued your triceps with the first two exercises, you might then do specific triceps exercises. This way you may effectively work out your triceps with less resistance and perhaps with fewer reps or sets. The same can be said for the seated leg press, leg extension, and leg curl machines, all of which exercise your thigh muscles. Similarly, the upper back machine and the lat-pull down machine primarily exercise your upper back and shoulders. But they also exercise and can pre-fatigue your biceps and the other muscles in the front of your arm. So using these machines prior to doing arm curls will allow you to get a good biceps workout with fewer arm curl exercises.

Variety

"After establishing a good level of fitness, you should endeavor to vary your workout to achieve even greater fitness and to avoid muscle boredom. Try different machines, different exercises, and different sequences of the exercises. You might alter the number of reps or sets and finish off with lightweight concentration reps. Do these very slowly while concentrating on tightening the muscle you're exercising. You might like the pec-deck to better isolate and exercise your chest muscles or the inner and outer thigh machines. Exercising the same muscles with different movements has the potential to further enhance the fitness of a muscle or group of muscles. However, for these first eight weeks, let's get fit on the ten important machines I've selected.

Review of the basic principles of strength training

"At the risk of being redundant, the basic principles on all of these machines are the same. While many programs vary in terms of reps and sets and the rate of progression, I'd like you to start by first determining your 'max':

Step 1 Establish the proper form, breathing technique, and the correct range of motion by doing the exercise or movement with no added resistance.

Step 2 Warm up your muscles by doing five reps with minimal resistance and rest for two and a half minutes.

Step 3 Increase the resistance, do another five reps and rest again for two and a half minutes.

Step 4 Try to max. See what the maximum amount of weight-resistance you can move through the exercise movement, in a one-time effort, with perfect form and without holding your breath. Rest again for two and a half minutes. Remember to use proper form and to keep breathing correctly.

"Now we are ready to start our resistance training program with the following steps:

Step 1 Use 75% of the max weight, to start your strength-training program and do five to eight reps for your first set with this resistance. Then rest for two and half minutes.

Step 2 Try to do a second and then a third set with this resistance, resting two and a half minutes between sets.

Step 3 Increase the number of reps to eight in each set and increase the number of sets to three.

Step 4 As your fitness improves, decrease the resting period between sets to an average of sixty seconds.

Step 5 The last rep of the last set should be the most difficult. If you feel you can do more, then increase the number of reps in each set to ten or twelve or more.

Step 6 When you can do three sets of twelve or more reps for four or more consecutive workouts, increase the weight resistance slightly and go back to doing eight reps for three sets.

Step 7 When you feel you have reached your goal, use this as your maintenance program for each exercise two to four times a week.

"Always remember the following ABCDs:

A—perfect form

B—good breathing technique

C—slower and lighter is better than quicker and heavier

D—progress gradually.

"Now, lads and lasses, let's get on these machines. Sheila, you take the seated shoulder press. Leonard, you get on the upper back machine; and Sam will take the seated bench press. Georgina and Joe, get everybody else on a machine.

The seated bench or chest press machine

"Let's go over here to Sam on the seated bench press machine [fig. 11C]. There are also recumbent bench press machines; but when I use a recumbent bench press, the blood rushes to my head and I get the feeling it's not so good for my blood pressure. So I don't recommend this machine for most of us, particularly us older folks. The seated bench press strengthens the pectoralis muscles—you know, your chest muscles. It also strengthens your shoulder muscles and your triceps. Those are the muscles in the back of your arms—the muscles that keep you from looking like you have a bag of grapes hanging back there.

"First, Sam, make sure you're positioned properly. I want you to be sure that your butt is back on the seat. Don't let it slide forward [fig. 11C wrong]. Your back should be straight and firmly positioned against the back support. Adjust the height of the seat so that the bench press handles are about the level of your nipples [fig. 11C correct]. Now do a few reps with no resistance other than the weight carrier so that you get the idea of the movement. Practice the proper form and breathing. For some of us, using

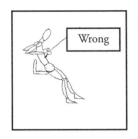
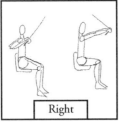

Fig 11C

the weight carrier without any added resistance may be all we need to start our resistance training. Again, this will vary from person to person and from machine to machine. Those of you on a pneumatic machine do the same thing without any pressure or weight-resistance.

"You'll note that on some of the newer versions of these seated bench press machines, your hands come closer together as you perform the positive phase of the rep. This adds an extra squeeze on your chest muscles and really improves the exercise. Now if you feel too much pressure on your shoulder joints when you start or when you return to the starting position, then adjust your range of motion in the exercise so that you don't stretch that far. It's better to do an exercise through a full range of motion, but not at the expense of injury. We can gradually improve our range of motion as our fitness improves.

The seated shoulder press machine

"Let's go over to Sheila on the seated shoulder press. This machine exercises the muscles of your shoulders, upper back, and triceps. Sheila also has to be sure to keep her butt back on the seat and her back firmly supported by the backrest [fig 11D].

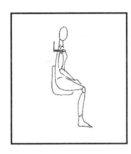
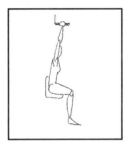

Fig 11D

"She should adjust the height of the seat so that the handle grips are at, or just above, her shoulders. As she raises the handles to perform the positive phase of each rep, she must be careful to avoid sliding her butt forward or leaning forward—to avoid jerking her back. When she extends her arms upward, she might feel discomfort in her shoulders or elbows. If that occurs, she should decrease the extension of her arms to a point just short of that.

"The same is true on the return to the starting position. Shorten the return to a point where little or no discomfort is felt in your elbows and shoulders. As we've said before, it's better to perform the exercise through a complete range of motion, but not at the expense of injury. You can gradually increase your range of motion by performing each exercise with that as one of your goals.

Triceps machine exercises

"There are three different triceps machines in this gym. As we said earlier, if you've pre-fatigued your triceps with the seated bench press or vertical shoulder press, now is a good time to do your triceps. The first machine uses an upper pulley attached to a triangular shaped bar [fig. 11E]. For this exercise, I want you to grasp the handles, keep your elbows tucked into your sides, and keep the point of the triangular bar just below your chin [fig. 11E right]. This is the starting position.

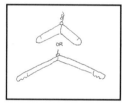

Fig 11E

"Now extend your arms slowly downward to do the positive phase of the rep and hold it for a count of one. Then slowly return to the starting position to complete the rep. The important things to remember in this exercise are to keep your back straight and to not let the point of the triangular bar rise above the height of your chin.

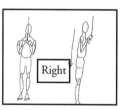

Fig 11E Right

"Some of us might try to bend our back and use our upper body weight to push the resistance downward [fig. 11E wrong]. Avoid this by fixing your feet about ten to twelve inches apart, keeping your elbows close to your body, tightening your abdominal muscles, and concentrating on not bending your back.

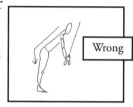

Fig 11E Wrong

"A slight bend in your knees can help avoid any strain on your back; but you have to fix that position. In other words, don't bend and straighten your knees while doing the exercise or you'll be using your body weight to move the resistance. Also, make sure the triangular bar has good grips or flanges or wear exercise gloves so that the bar doesn't slip out of your hands and pop you one in the chin. A slight variation of this exercise can be done using a straight bar. Try to do these triceps exercises slowly; and use light resistance so that you can concentrate on tightening the triceps muscles and avoid compromising your form.

"Some other very good triceps exercises are the seated arm extension apparatus and the dip machine. And again, variation between machines can avoid muscle boredom and enhance the fitness of your muscles. There are also excellent floor exercises for the triceps as well as triceps exercises that can be done with dumbbells. But we'll get into that later.

The upper back machine

"Now, let's go over to Leonard on the upper back machine. This is a fantastic exercise. It's a pulling exercise. It exercises your mid and upper back muscles, your shoulders, and arms. These back muscles are big; and exercising them can burn a lot of calories."

"I've been waiting for you, Doc. In fact, I'm all pooped out waiting for you," joked Leonard.

"Okay," Zinney responded. "Let's get it on. You'll note that Leonard is positioned in such a way that he's facing the machine and that his chest is firmly placed against a padded support.

"Also, note that there are two sets of handles on the machine. One set is horizontal and one set is vertical. The height of the seat should be adjusted so that the horizontal handles are about the level of his nipples."

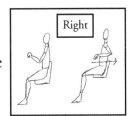

Fig 11F Right

"In my case, that would be about the same level as my bellybutton," Miriam chuckled.

"Good point, Miriam. So instead, you'd position the horizontal handles below your shoulders and level with the upper part of your chest." said Zinney. "Now using the horizontal handles will work more of the higher upper back; and using the vertical handles will get more of the mid to upper back muscles. Again, this is a pulling exercise. The exercise is performed by extending your arms, grasping the handles, and pulling against the resistance—pulling towards you [fig. 11F right]. You use the padded chest plate for support.

"To do this correctly, sit with your chest firmly placed against the chest support. If you come away from the chest support or off the seat, you're doing it incorrectly. You're using your legs and straining your low back [fig. 11F wrong]. You don't want to do that.

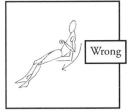

Fig 11F Wrong

The lat pull down

"The lat bar or upper pull down bar is another pulling exercise for your upper back, shoulders, and arms. The positive phase of the rep consists of pulling the bar down to a point that is level with your upper chest [fig. 11G];

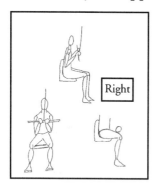

Right

Fig 11G

and the negative phase entails returning the bar to the starting position. You can use this instead of the upper back machine or alternate between the two. If you use a wide grip on the lat bar and do the pull down exercise behind your neck and across the back of your shoulders, you can exercise your lower lat muscles."

"What are the 'lat muscles'? You keep referring to a lat bar and lat muscles and I don't know what they are," said Sheila.

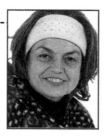

"Those are those big beautiful muscles in your back that give bodybuilders a terrific 'V' shape to their torso,"

Zinney answered. "They're called the latismus dorsi muscles or lats for short. Using the lat pull down bar behind your back can really work these out and get them big. But that's not what most of you are here for. While some trainers might encourage your using a wide grip and doing the pull down behind your back, I'm a little concerned about that. It puts a lot of strain on the shoulder joints; and a lot of us aren't flexible enough to do this without getting hurt.

"However, you can get a very good workout by using a closer grip and doing the pull downs in front of your chest. You can do alternating sets with your palms facing forwards and with your palms facing backwards. You can get a great workout of your upper back, shoulders, and arms this way.

"There are some additional tips I'd like to share with you. Adjust the height of the seat so that when you grip the bar, there is a very slight bend in your elbows. Whether your palms are facing forward or backward, grip the bar so that there's about ten to twelve inches between your hands. This is a good starting position for this exercise. You can vary this as you become accustomed to the exercise.

"Keep your feet flat and don't come off the seat. People have a tendency to jerk off the seat in this exercise. When they do this in the positive phase, they're using their body weight to get the resistance moving. If they do it in the negative phase, they're also reducing the effectiveness of the exercise. Some of these machines have a padded support bar that goes across the top of your knees. This can help to keep you from rising up during the exercise.

"Do the exercise slowly to a count of four and hold for a count of one between the positive and negative phases of the movement. And another thing, make sure your grip is firm and use exercise gloves so that the bar doesn't slip from your sweaty hands and pop you a shot in the kisser.

"All that having been said, there is another variation of this machine that I prefer more than the lat bar. It's a pull down machine that has both horizontal and vertical handles. Using this version, you can vary the position and width of your grip.

Arm curl machine

"Now that we've pre-fatigued our arms with the upper back machine or the lat pull machine, let's go over to the arm curl machine [fig. 11H]. This machine exercises the muscles in the front of your upper arms like your biceps. It can also improve your grip and forearm muscles. It's very important that you adjust the seat so that

the back of your upper arms rest comfortably on the padded supports. When you grip the handles, there should be a slight bend in your elbows and the padded chest support should be flush against your torso. Keep it that way throughout the exercise.

"This will keep you from coming off your seat or from leaning forward or backward [fig. 11H wrong] during the exercise. If you do, you will be using your back and your legs to help you move the resistance instead of your biceps—so sit tight.

"The positive phase of the rep consists of flexing your arms against the resistance; and the negative phase consists of returning to the starting position [fig. 11H right]. No other part of your body should change position. If you use an underhand grip, this exercise should concentrate its effort on the biceps. If you use an overhand grip, you can exercise some of the other muscles in your arm, like the brachialis muscle. Do these arm curls slowly, to the count of four and hold for the count of one. Sit tight and concentrate on good breathing. There are also some really great arm exercises we can do with dumbbells, which we'll get to later.

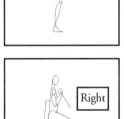

Fig 11H

The seated leg press

"Next, let's talk about our best fat burners—our legs. The muscles in our thighs and legs are huge and strong. Exercising them can burn a lot of calories, increase the mineral density of our bones, and increase our strength. All of this adds up to better balance, more endurance, and less chance of falls and fractures. But be aware that these exercises put strain on the knee and hip joints. This can be good or it can be bad. If you've had orthopedic problems or surgery in these areas, it's important to check with your doctor as to what exercises he or she thinks would be appropriate for you.

"The classic exercise used by weightlifters to build strong legs is known as squats. That's where the weightlifter does deep knee bends with a weight-loaded barbell across his shoulders. It's a great exercise for building huge, strong thighs; but may not be so good for us folks. It puts an enormous amount of strain on your knee joints, back, and shoulders. The deeper the squat, the better the exercise, but also greater the risk of injury. That's why I think most people are better served by using the seated leg press machine [fig. 11I] where we can isolate the exercise to these leg muscles and reduce the risk of injury.

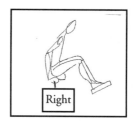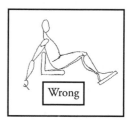

Fig 11I

"In using this machine, it's important to sit so that your butt is back on the seat with your knees bent, your feet flat and placed firmly on the resistance pedals. Your toes should be pointing straight and your head bent forward. This is the starting position. The positive phase of each rep is performed by straightening your legs against the resistance. The negative phase is performed by returning to the starting position. If you slide forward, you might strain your back [fig. 11I wrong]. Keeping your head bent forward can help reduce strain on your back. Here too, the deeper you flex those thighs the better the exercise but the greater the likelihood of hurting your knee or hip joints.

"Only use a range of motion that's comfortable and don't increase the resistance too quickly. You can dramatically increase your leg strength with this exercise without exceeding your comfort zone. Do this by gradually increasing the number of reps, sets, and resistance and gradually increasing the degree of flexion as your comfort permits. There's no rush. Remember our motto: Strain a little, Gain a lot.

192

"You can further strengthen your thigh muscles by slightly altering the position of your feet for a few reps or sets. If you point your toes slightly inward, you will put a little more strain on the muscles of your outer thigh. If you point your toes outward, you will give more exercise to the muscles of your inner thigh. Doing a few reps or sets this way can help to round out the development of your thigh muscles.

Strengthening your calf muscles

"You can also exercise your calf muscles with this machine. As you know, the leg press is done with your feet flat on the resistance pedals. Keeping the balls and heels of your feet flush with the resistance pedals helps to incorporate the muscles in both the front (the quadriceps) and back of your thigh (the hamstrings) during the exercise. But if you push the resistance with the balls of your feet, with your heels raised up and off the pedals for a few reps or sets, you will also exercise your calf muscles.

"You can even isolate the exercise to the muscles in the back of your calf with this machine by doing sets of heel raises with your knees straight. With your legs straight, push against the resistance with the balls of your feet so that you push the resistance

away from your heels, so that your heels rise up from the pedals. Do this slowly and then return your heels slowly to the resistance pedals. As you repeat this, you will feel your calf muscles getting pumped up. There are also other machines and floor exercises to strengthen your calf muscles; but we'll go over them later.

The seated leg extension

"Now that we've pre-fatigued the muscles in our thighs, we can do some strength training that will focus on the front of our thighs (the quadriceps) with the leg extension machine. You'll note that there is a seat and two sets of rollers [fig. 11J] on this machine, both of which can be adjusted to your size and the length of your legs. Miriam is sitting on the machine with her knees bent over the upper set of rollers and the front of her feet behind the lower set of rollers.

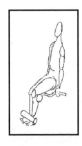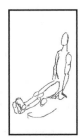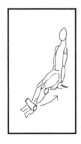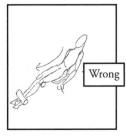

Fig 11J

"This is the starting position for this exercise. Note how she sits back on the seat. Her back is flush against the support.

"There is a handle on each side of the seat that she can grasp to stabilize and secure this position. The positive phase of the rep consists of slowly straightening her legs against the resistance and holding for a count of one; and the negative phase consists of slowly returning to the starting position. She's going to do three sets of ten reps each and rest for 45 seconds between each set. It's really important that she doesn't slide forward on the seat [fig. 11J wrong]. If she does, she will be straining her low back during the exercise.

"This is a fabulous exercise for strengthening and defining those muscles in the front of your thighs, the quadriceps. You might get even better definition by concentrating on the muscle contraction as you straighten your legs; and also by holding it out there for a longer count between the positive and negative phases of some or all of the reps. As in the leg press, you might vary the direction of your feet for one or more reps or sets inwards or outwards. This can further exercise the muscles on the outer and inner thighs.

Keiser Leg Curl Machine

The seated leg curl

"The seated leg curl is a fabulous exercise for the muscles in the back of your thigh—your hamstrings. These muscles play an important role in walking, running, stair climbing, and maintaining balance. Most of the leg exercises we do and most of our activities exercise the quadriceps—the muscles in the front of our thighs. As a result, our quadriceps muscles get much stronger than our hamstrings. For better balance, we would like our hamstrings to be about two-thirds as strong as our quadriceps; but in most of us, they're not even close. This imbalance in strength, together with a failure to do proper stretching, is responsible for a lot of falls and injuries. I'm sure many of you have heard of professional athletes who were sidelined because of a pulled hamstring.

"You'll note that this machine also has two padded plates. Place your knees beneath the padded plate closest to you and your feet on top of the extended plate. The seat and other parts of the machine can be adjusted to accommodate your size. Sit back on the seat with legs extended and a slight bend at your knees. Your back should be flush against the back support. Keep a firm grip on the handles to help fix your position. This is the starting position for this exercise.

194

"The positive phase of the rep is performed as you bend and slowly curl your legs backward. The negative phase is performed as you return to the starting position. Here again, the exercise is done slowly and with perfect form. Try to do three sets of eight reps with about one minute rest between sets. It will take a little time, but we're all going to get there.

"There are a number of different machines to exercise hamstrings besides this one. I like the seated variety because it offers more protection against back strain. But whatever hamstring exercises you do, please don't forget to stretch these muscles when you're done.

The abdominal muscles

"Next, let's talk about exercising our abdominal muscles or what are commonly referred to as our 'abs.' A lot of people don't realize the importance of these muscles. They think exercising them is only for the purpose of producing a sexy-looking washboard appearance to their belly. Not so! The abs assist you in breathing, in having bowel movements, and, of even greater importance, in maintaining the integrity of your low back. Weak abs not only predispose you to hernias; but they let your potbelly protrude more so that it pulls on your low back.

"On the other hand, well-conditioned and strong abs counterbalance your stronger back muscles, producing greater stability to your low back. One of the most effective ways of preventing or alleviating low back problems is to condition your abdominal muscles. You will be amazed at how much better you will feel and how much better your back will feel when you strengthen these muscles. While less important, a marvelous side benefit can be a slimmer and more attractive appearance. Having said this, let's get on with the exercise.

The abdominal crunch machine

"Floor exercises to strengthen the abdominal muscles are among my favorites and we'll get into them a little later. However, the abdominal crunch machine can also produce a magnificent abdominal workout. It can be used as an alternative or as an addition to floor exercises; and it's particularly useful for people who have difficulty getting up or down from the floor. Joe has been kind enough to volunteer his services for this demonstration, so let's have at it.

"As you can see, Joe is facing a padded chest support with his feet firmly anchored behind two stationary foot supports [fig. 11K].

"The seat is adjusted to fit his size so that the upper level of the support is

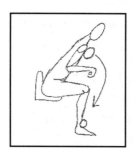

Fig 11K

about the level of his upper chest. His feet are flat on the floor and comfortably but firmly positioned behind the stationary foot supports. His hands and arms are taken out of the movement by placing them firmly on the handles. This is the starting position for this exercise.

"The positive phase of each rep consists of bending forward and squeezing and crunching the abdominal muscles into contraction. The negative phase consists of returning to the starting position. Do both phases of this exercise slowly; and squeeze the contraction between the positive and negative phase for a count of three or four.

"Some of us will do better with three sets of eight to fifteen or more reps using light resistance, and others will feel they've gotten a better workout with fewer reps and more resistance. Here again, there's some bending in this exercise. If you've had hip surgery, check with your doctor before doing it.

"Ok! Let's all of us get going on these machines. Joe, Georgina, Raul, and I will supervise your journey into a new and better world. When we're all done, we're not done—not until we've done our stretching. Remember: if you stretch for life, you might stretch your life.

Very slow weight lifting

"Before leaving this subject, I ought to tell you there are some advocates of even slower exercise repetitions than I've recommended. Some experts have recommended that each repetition be a fourteen second rep—seven seconds in the active direction and seven in the return phase of the exercise. This kind of program usually involves doing only one set of five reps of each movement once a week as a total workout.

"While there is some evidence that this can significantly increase muscle mass, it requires a lot of concentration and seems to encourage breath holding. Advocates claim it is safer and more effective. While this may work for some folks, I think the jury is still out on these issues. And I have very serious concerns in regard to the health benefits of only exercising once a week.

Concentric and eccentric muscle contraction

"However, as all of you know, I am an advocate of doing your resistance training with slow reps as we've described. It decreases the chance of muscle injury and increases the rate of muscle development. When you are lifting weight, your muscle is contracting, or shortening. This is *concentric* muscle contraction. When you are slowly lowering the weight, your muscle is contracted against resistance as it is lengthening. This is *eccentric* muscle contraction. Since you can lower more weight than you can lift, you might improve your muscle mass and bone strength even more effectively by prolonging the return phase of each rep. So, if you feel you have to decrease the length of time of the positive phase of your reps (concentric contraction), try to prolong the return phase (eccentric contraction). For example, you might do your reps with a two or three second positive phase and a six or seven second return phase. After you've achieved a modicum of fitness, you might get the best of that other world by doing the last one or two reps of each set at a very slow rate.

"The day after next, we're going to come back here for another workout. When we're finished with that, we'll get a chance to show you some strength training and balance exercises that you can do here or at home. Tomorrow, rest those muscles. Do your stretching and maybe a little walking. Let's all of us have a good one and we'll all look forward to our next meeting at 10:00 A.M. sharp the day after tomorrow. Bye, all."

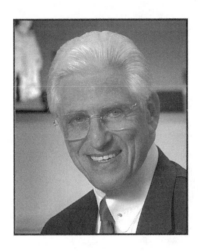

12

Your balance is improved
And your agility grooved,
If you just take a seat
And repeat and repeat.

Strength and Balance Exercises You Can Do at Home

The group was ushered into an unused racketball court with mats and chairs spread around the room. Zinney began, "I know that some of you simply can't get to the gym on a regular basis for one of many reasons. Others might prefer to continue strength and balance training at home after you've learned how to train in the gym. Some of you might even want to develop a gym at home. As I've said before, many manufacturers produce excellent strength training equipment (Keiser, Cybex, Bowflex, etc.) that can be used to furnish a gym at home. There are also a variety of treadmills and stationary bikes on the market for cardiopulmonary conditioning. But not to worry. There are also excellent strength training, balance training, and endurance exercises that you can do at home without a lot of fancy equipment. Some of the strength exercises we will do with dumbells, as well as the balance exercises, are so important that we should all practice them regardless of where we workout—at home or in the gym. The equipment you need is very little: a chair, floor space, a couple pairs of dumbbells, and ankle weights. Instead of dumbbells, you can use plastic half-gallon containers that have handles. By filling them with varying amounts of water or sand, you can change the weight resistance for different exercises and use them like dumbbells. Ankle weights, which you can buy in almost any sporting goods store, would be of additional benefit; but they're not essential.

Principles of training

"The principles and precautions in regard to resistance training at home are the same as those we would use in the gym. At the risk of being redundant, we'll review some of them here

199

because they're so very important. You should do a set of eight to fifteen repetitions (reps) of each movement with perfect form.

"Gradually work towards doing two or three sets of each exercise and, as you progress, shorten the rest period between sets from two and one half minutes to 60 seconds or less. Start slowly, using minimal resistance at first.

"When you find you can easily do three sets of an exercise with sixty-second rest periods between sets, increase the number of reps in each set to ten and then to twelve or fifteen. When you can do two or three sets of twelve to fifteen reps in each set with sixty-second rest periods between sets, you're ready to advance. Increase the weight or resistance slightly and go back to eight reps in each set. Then again, increase the number of reps per set gradually.

"Continuing this progressive process will challenge your muscles and cause them to get stronger. It will also increase your endurance for repetitive motion. Some of us may not be able to do eight reps of an exercise yet. Well, an old Chinese says, 'Every journey begins by taking the first step.' If you can't do eight reps, do two or three reps. Gradually try to increase your ability. If you try, and if you stay with it, you will improve.

"Breathe in at the starting position of each repetition and breathe out against the resistance. Then, fill your lungs with air during the return to the starting position. Repeat this sequence of inhaling and exhaling with each rep. Stretch the muscles you've exercised between sets or at least before going on to the next kind of movement. And remember to do your stretching exercises every day, even on days that you don't do resistance or endurance training.

Frequency

"You'll recall from our prior discussions that exercise stimulates all of the magnificent biological mechanisms that make your muscles grow and become stronger. And you also know that your muscles grow and increase in strength while they're resting and not while you're exercising them. So, if you're going to strength train every day, alternate the muscle groups that you workout. For example, you can do your upper body on Monday, Wednesday, and Friday and your lower body muscles on Tuesday, Thursday, and Saturday. I'll let you rest a little on Sunday. If you're going to strength train only two or three days a week, then exercise both your upper and lower body muscles the same days.

"Recent studies suggest that if we increase the intensity and duration of our workout, most of us older folks can probably do as well by strength training twice a week. If you use this schedule, I suggest something like Tuesday and Friday strength training sessions. This permits one forty-eight hour rest period and one seventy-two hour rest period between resistance exercise sessions. In some of us, this added period of rest promotes muscle growth and strength. It also allows more time for endurance training on the other days. These are the principles that apply to the exercises we're now going to demonstrate.

Chair stand

"Let's start with the lower body. Our leg strength is extremely important in maintaining balance and preventing falls. In this regard, all of the muscles in our legs play an important role. The chair stand exercise involves most of these muscles and is one of the more important exercises in this regard. Let's get Sam up here to demonstrate this movement."

"Me again?" said Sam. "Can't you pick on someone else, Doc, at least once in a while?"

"I've 'picked' on other people, Sam," Zinney replied. "It's just that you're such a good subject and so coopera-

tive. So c'mon over here. And let's sit down to shape up."

Sam, more happily than he would have people believe, sat in the chair in the middle of the room and sighed. "Ok, Doc, I'm ready."

"As all of you can see, there's a pillow placed behind the small of Sam's back for some support. We want Sam to go from sitting up straight to standing up straight without leaning his shoulders too far forward. Do it slowly to the count of three [fig. 12A].

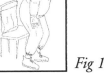

Fig 12A

"Then, sit back down again, slowly to the count of three. That's what I mean when I say 'Sit down to Shape up and Repeat and Repeat and Repeat.' Do a set of eight to fifteen reps, then rest and do another set or two. Some of us may have to use our hands to help us with this movement, but the idea is to improve our performance of this exercise to where we don't have to use our hands at all.

"It's important to keep your back straight and avoid jerking motions. Also, you'll find this exercise more difficult to perform if you use a chair that has a low seat. Start with a chair that has a high seat; and if the exercise becomes easy, then you can switch to a chair with a lower seat. If your chair is too low for you at the start, you can raise the height of the seat by adding a firm cushion. When and if this exercise becomes too easy for you, you can increase the resistance by performing the same exercise while holding dumbbells or a telephone book.

Knee extension and dorsi-flexion of the foot

"Next, Sam is going to demonstrate the leg extension exercise. This movement will strengthen the muscles in the front of the thigh known as the quadriceps and also, the muscles of your shin in the front of your lower leg. It's important that while sitting in the chair, your feet hang freely or that only the balls of your feet or your toes touch the floor. You can do this by sitting up straight and placing some rolled up towels on the chair under your knees or by raising the seat with a firm cushion. If you need to, support yourself by placing your hands on the sides of the seat near the front.

"Now, extend one leg slowly for three seconds. Hold it out there for three seconds while flexing and squeezing your foot and toes towards your head during the hold [fig. 12B].

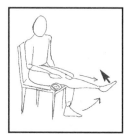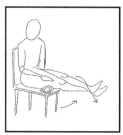

Fig 12B

202

"Then lower your leg back to the starting position—slowly to the count of three seconds. Do two or three sets of eight to twelve reps each—first with one leg then with the other. As your confidence increases, you might be able to do both legs at one time; and then when your strength increases, it will be time to buy some ankle weights. You might vary this exercise by crossing your feet and squeezing your thighs together when your legs are extended like a scissors movement [fig. 12B]. This will also help to exercise some of the muscles of the inner thighs."

"Doc, what's the reason for flexing the foot upwards during the hold part of the movement?" Leonard asked.

"It helps to strengthen the muscles of your shin, the front of your lower leg. This group of muscles is referred to as the dorsi-flexors of the foot because they flex the foot upward. When those muscles are weak, your step gets sloppy. Your toes and the ball of your foot tend to drag when you bring your foot forward. This can increase the likelihood of shuffling, stumbling, and tripping. These muscles not only help you walk, they help you climb stairs and take your foot off the gas pedal to place it on the brake.

"So when you have your knee extended and your foot flexed upwards toward you, concentrate and squeeze those muscles in the front of your shin, the dorsi-flexors of the foot. Few people exercise these muscles. But it's a good idea. They're more important than most people realize in maintaining balance and agility, to avoiding tripping. As an added benefit, this movement also helps to stretch the muscles in the back of your calf."

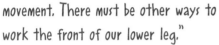

"I find that part of the exercise awkward," said Sam. "I'd rather just concentrate on the front of my thighs with this movement. There must be other ways to work the front of our lower leg."

"Surely," said Zinney. "Here's one I like. Sit in the chair with your feet flat on the floor. Keep your heels on the floor while you raise the balls of your feet upwards and off the floor and curl your toes towards your head [fig. 12C]. Hold it and squeeze it for three seconds. Do two or three sets of eight to fifteen reps each. If that becomes too easy for you, you can hold telephone books or dumbbells on your knees to add resistance.

"Let's move on now to some of the exercises you can do while standing behind the chair. There's a whole series of them that can be done in sequence to give you a great workout. Ok, Sam, stand behind the chair.

Calf muscle and ankle muscle exercises

"We just finished exercising the front of our lower legs, now we'll work the backs—our calf muscles. Support yourself by holding onto the back of the chair and start with your feet flat on the floor.

"To the slow count of three, raise up on the balls of your feet, on your tippy, tippy toes, and hold it for one second. Then slowly lower yourself back to the starting position, also to the count of three seconds. Do two or three sets of about eight to fifteen reps in each. This exercise will strengthen the muscles of your calf and your ankle. When it gets easy, try it with one leg at a time [fig. 12D].

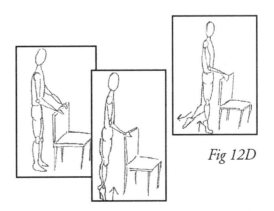

Fig 12D

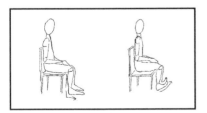

Fig 12C

203

Knee flexion exercise for the back of your thigh

"The next exercise that Sam will demonstrate will strengthen the muscles in the back of your thigh. They're called the hamstring muscles. Using the same position and supporting yourself by holding onto the back of the chair, bend one leg backwards and upwards [fig. 12E] so that the heel of your foot comes as close to the back of your thigh as possible.

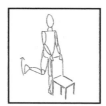

Fig 12E

"Again, do this slowly to the count of three or four seconds and hold it there for a second. Then slowly return to the starting position to the count of three or four seconds. Do two or three sets of eight to fifteen reps with each leg. Alternate your legs for each set. When this or any of the leg or hip exercises become easy to do, add ankle weights.

Hip flexion

"Sam, now let's go to the hip flexion movement. I believe that strengthening the muscles that flex your hips is another important exercise that prevents shuffling and falls. While many gyms have excellent machines for this exercise, you can do it at home. As you progress, add ankle weights to further enhance your strength. While standing off to the side of the chair and using the back of the chair for support, bend your knee upward toward your abdomen as far as you can [fig. 12F].

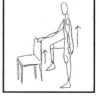

Fig 12F

"It's important that you stand straight, don't bend your back. Do this slowly to the count of three or four seconds and hold it for a second and then slowly return to the starting position. Do one set of eight to fifteen reps with each leg, then try another one or two sets.

Side leg raise

"Ok, Sam. Now let's do the side leg raise. This exercise strengthens the muscles on the outer thighs and hips. Stand directly behind the chair and support yourself by holding the back of the chair. Keep your back and your legs straight as you raise one leg outward and toward the side about six to twelve inches [fig. 12G].

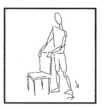

Fig 12G

"Do this slowly to the count of three or four seconds and hold it out there for a count of one second. Then, slowly return to the starting position. Do one set of eight to fifteen reps with each leg then do another one or two more sets.

Hip extension

"Alright, Sam, this is your last chance at being a celebrity here—the hip extension exercise. This exercise will strengthen the muscles of your buttocks and your low back muscles. Stand about a foot or a little more behind the chair with your feet about six to twelve inches apart. Support yourself with your hands on the back of the chair [fig. 12H].

"Bend slightly forward at the hips, not at the waist. This is the starting position for this movement. Raise one

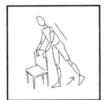

Fig 12H

leg straight back but keep the leg straight. Don't bend your knee or point your toes. Raise your leg slowly to the count of three or four seconds, hold it for one second, then slowly return to the starting position. Do one set of eight to fifteen reps with each leg, then repeat one or two more sets.

Upper body strength training at home

"John, we're now ready for your act. You're going to be our celebrity demonstrator for some movements and then we'll have lovely Miriam take the spotlight for some others."

John happily took a seat in the front of the room, flexed his biceps, and, to everyone's amusement, said:

"It's no surprise
That if you exercise,
You'll get hard
When you strip some lard."

"That's pretty good! I may use that," said Zinney. "The first set of exercises that John will demonstrate consists of three movements aimed at strengthening the muscles of the shoulder girdle. They are best performed with dumbbells; but as I said earlier, plastic half-gallon jugs or bags of sand can be used instead of dumbbells.

"Please note, your position in the chair is very important. Sit in the chair with your back straight and your feet flat on the floor. Spread your feet so that they are about as far apart as your shoulders and hold a dumbbell in each hand. Now you're ready to start the first movement.

"With each exercise, start with a weight that is light enough for you to do eight to fifteen reps in each set with perfect form and with 60-second rest periods between each set. When you can do two sets of twelve to fifteen reps, increase the weight slightly, and go back to eight reps. Then when you can do twelve reps with the new weight, you can increase the weight again. As you get stronger, you can gradually increase the weight; but not until you can do two sets of twelve to fifteen reps.

Side arm-raise

"This exercise will strengthen the muscles of the side of your shoulder girdle. With a dumbbell in each hand, your palms facing inward and your arms straight, slowly raise your arms upwards on each side until they are about the level of your shoulders [fig. 12I]. Raise your arms to the count of three, hold it for a second, then slowly return to the starting position. Very good, John. Let's go on.

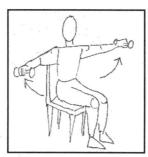

Fig 12I

Forward arm-raise

"This exercise will strengthen the muscles of the front of the shoulder girdle. Start with your arms down at your sides and your palms facing backward. Raise both arms upward to shoulder height with your palms facing backward. Alternatively, you can rotate your hands as you raise your arms so that your palms are facing upward; but don't bend too much at the elbows [fig. 12J]. Do it slowly to the count of three, hold it, then slowly return to the starting position.

Fig 12J

Vertical Rows

"The vertical row movement is a fabulous exercise to strengthen the muscles of your upper back (the trapezious muscles), your neck muscles, and the muscles of your shoulder girdle. This exercise will also help to strengthen and pre-fatigue the muscles of the front of your arms in preparation for the next group of exercises to be discussed (curls). They can be done standing or sitting. Here's how: With a dumbell in each hand and your palms facing backwards, pull the dumbells straight up to the level of your upper chest so that your elbows are pointing out [fig. 12K]. Do it slowly, without jerking your arms or your back. Hold it for a second or two and then slowly lower your hands to

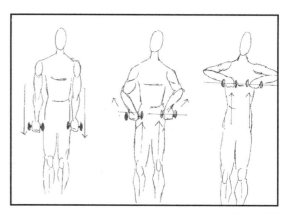

Fig 12K

the starting position. Try one to three sets of eight to twelve reps.

"Now it's Miriam's chance to be our celebrity. C'mon up here, Miriam. And tell us, Miriam, do you have a little ditty to match John's?"

Miriam gracefully took the chair in the front of the room, and then said, "Yes, indeed I do. It goes like this:

"A pound of muscle,
You'll soon discern,
Shrinks your bustle
And the fat you spurn.

"Now I'm ready, Doc. So push my starter button." Zinney carefully inspected her position to make sure that she was sitting straight and that both feet were flat on the floor and spread slightly inside her shoulders.

Zinney continued, "Ok, folks, the series of movements Miriam is going to demonstrate will strengthen the muscles in the front of our upper arms and also our forearms. Here again, I suggest you try to do one set of eight reps of each of these exercises in sequence, one after the other with a 60-second rest period between each set. Remember to avoid swinging the dumbbells. Now, for the first exercise.

Twist curls

"With your palms facing inward and a dumbbell in each hand, slowly bend your arms upwards at the elbow while turning your hands so that the palms of your hands point towards the front of your shoulders [fig. 12L].

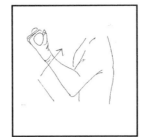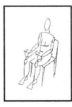

Fig 12L

"As with the other exercises we've demonstrated, do this movement slowly to the count of three seconds, hold for one second, then slowly return to the starting position.

"A very important aspect of the arm curl exercises that Miriam is demonstrating is to keep your elbows firmly tucked into your sides during the entire movement. Don't lean forward or jerk or swing the weight upwards. If you do, you'll be using your back and your shoulder muscles to raise the weight instead of isolating the exercise to the arm muscles. You won't get the full benefit of the exercise. You can do this movement while standing, but you are less likely to 'cheat' by doing the exercise in a seated position. When you have finished a set of eight to ten reps of the twist curls, rest 45 to 60 seconds; and then do another one or two sets.

Traditional curls

"If you really want to develop sharp looking biceps, you can try a set or two of traditional curls. Let me explain as Miriam demonstrates the movements. Start with the dumbbells at your side and the palms of your hands facing forward. There's no twisting in this movement. With your palms facing forward and your hands at your sides, flex your arms all the way upward so that your palms are facing the front of your shoulders. Remember to keep your elbows tucked closely against your body throughout these movements. Do the movement slowly to the count of three seconds and hold it for a second while concentrating on the squeeze. Then slowly return to the starting position. Do eight to twelve repetitions and rest for sixty seconds. Do another set or two and then try a set or two of reverse curls. This is basically the same movement but done with your palms facing backwards.

Reverse curls

"With your palms facing backwards, bend your arms upwards at the elbow so that the backs of your hands are facing the fronts of your shoulders. Again, do it slowly to the count of three or four seconds, hold it for a second and then slowly return to the starting position. Try to do eight to ten reps and then rest for about 60 seconds. Then try another set or two if you like.

"Ok, Miriam, you did great. We've really worked out the front of our arms. Now let's go on. The next set of exercises will be to strengthen the back part of our arms. Craig, it's your turn to be our celebrity demonstrator."

"I'll be glad to," said Craig. "But I don't have any ditties—just great performance."

"That's all we need," said Zinney. "So switch chairs with your wife and let's get it on.

Triceps extension

"There are several very good exercises you can do at home to strengthen the muscles in the back of your arms. The one that uses dumbbells is called the 'triceps extension' and it's so good that you should do it here in the gym as well.

"Position yourself slightly towards the front of the seat with your feet about one foot apart. Hold the dumbbell in one hand with your palm facing inward and bend your arm so that the weight hangs over and behind your shoulder. Immobilize and support the upper part of this arm with your other hand. This is the starting position.

"Now, slowly lift the weight straight up towards the ceiling to the count of three, then slowly return to the starting position [fig. 12M]. Keep your back straight throughout the movement and concentrate on keeping the

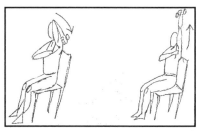

Fig 12M

upper part of your arm still. Do a set of eight to fifteen reps, then do a set with the other arm. Take a 45 to 60 second rest, before repeating the exercise with each arm.

Shoulder press

"Another good exercise for your arms also strengthens the muscles of the shoulder girdle. Hoist the dumbbells to shoulder height and hold them with your palms facing inward. This is the starting position for this movement. Now, straighten your arms by

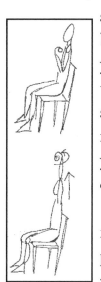

Fig 12N

slowly lifting the dumb bells straight up over your head. As you lift them, rotate your hands so that your palms are facing forward when your arms have been completely extended [fig. 12N]. Then slowly return to the starting position. Again, do about eight to fifteen reps, rest a minute, then

try another set or two. Alternatively, you can work one arm at a time or alternate arms.

The chair dip

"This exercise strengthens your muscles in the back of your arms as well as some of your chest and shoulder muscles. You need a chair with sturdy armrests. When you sit in the chair, the armrests should be slightly higher then your waist. If the armrests are too high, then use a cushion; but if they're too low, use a different chair. Place your hands on the armrests just slightly towards the front of your waist and lean forward a little.

"Keep your back straight and lift yourself off the seat by straightening your arms [fig. 12O]. Do this to the

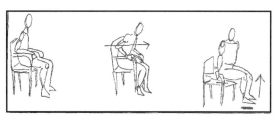

Fig 12O

slow count of three and hold it for the count of one. Then slowly lower yourself into the seat. Try to do eight to twelve reps, then rest for a minute. Try to do several sets. Many of you may not have the strength to do this exercise without using your legs to help you. That's ok. As your strength increases, you can try to use your legs less and less, then not at all.

Push-ups

"Push-ups are among the most popular floor exercises used to strengthen the muscles in the back of the arms, the triceps, and also the chest muscles. They can be very hard for some of us who haven't exercised for a long time; but there are modifications of the exercise that many of us will find useful. Let's first demonstrate the classic push-up before showing you the modifications that most of us can use. Craig, don't get worried. I'm gonna give you a rest and demonstrate these myself.

"The classic push-up is done off the floor with the hands placed at shoulder level. Slowly lower and raise your body [fig. 12P]. You can strengthen different aspects of the musculature by varying the position of your hands—placing them further apart, closer together, or higher than shoulder level. Some athletes even do them on their fingertips or even on one-hand.

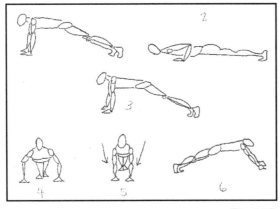

Fig 12P

All fours modified floor push-ups

"Many of us will be able to do a modified push-up by positioning ourselves on all fours, on our hands and knees. Place your hands about three to six inches in front of your shoulders with your arms straight. Keep your hands spread about as wide apart as your shoulders. This is the starting position for this exercise.

"Lower your chest slowly to the floor [fig. 12Q] and then use your arms to lift yourself back to the starting position. You can vary this position by putting your hands directly under your shoulders and moving your knees back three to six inches. As your strength improves, vary the position of your hands and knees, increase the number of repetitions, and possibly progress to full floor push-ups. However, if all-fours is too strenuous, try wall push-ups.

Wall push-ups

"Doing push-ups against the wall is a modification that most of us will be able to do. Stand at arm's length facing the wall so that your fingertips can

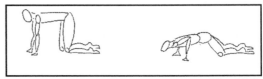

Fig 12Q

just about touch the wall. Lean forward so that the palms of your hands are flush with the wall and support yourself with straight arms and a straight back. This is the starting position for this movement.

"Now slowly bend your arms so that your face and your upper chest become almost flush with the wall [fig. 12R]; and then, slowly return to

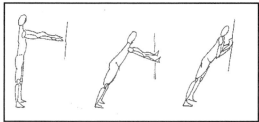

Fig 12R

the starting position. Do a set of three, five, or any number up to fifteen. Rest for about a minute and repeat the exercise. Then gradually increase the number of reps. When it becomes easy, you can try the modified floor push-ups on all fours.

Abdominal muscle exercises

"The next exercises we're going to discuss are the ways we can strengthen our abdominal muscles. These muscles are extremely important to maintaining a healthy low back and abdomen. They're important to breathing and to other normal daily living activities—such as the simple, or sometimes not so simple, act of having a bowel movement. We've already demonstrated the use of the abdominal crunch machines in the gym. Now we're going to show you how to exercise these muscles at home. Leonard is very good at this and I'm going to ask him to come up here and go through the movements for us as I describe them.

"Then I'll come around and check all of you out as you try them yourselves. The first kind of ab exercises we'll discuss are concentration exercises.

Concentration Abs

"Concentration abs can be done standing, sitting, or lying on your back. Let's try the standing one first. Stand with your back flush against the wall [fig. 12S].

"Now, suck in your abdomen. Think of the front of your abdomen moving back against your spine. Squeeze it in for a second or two, then relax. Do it again a little harder, then relax. Do two or three sets of five to thirty reps. Squeezing longer and harder can produce better results than more numerous rapid squeezes. You can do the same exercise while lying on your back or even sitting in a chair.

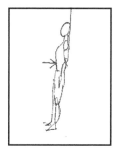

Fig 12S

Using the chair, you can do them at work, at a meeting, or at home while watching TV; and no one will even realize you're working out."

"Oh, I don't know about that," John chuckled. "Look at our screwed up expressions and red faces when we're doing this. Anyone watching would be sure that we're passing gas—or something more substantive."

"You've got a point there," laughed Zinney as he surveyed the room. "I guess if you folks are gonna do this in public, you're gonna have to learn to control your facial expressions.

Crunches

"Let's move on now to abdominal crunches you can do on the floor. An exercise mat would be helpful, but it's not essential. A soft carpet or towel is just as good.

"The classic exercise for abs is the 'sit-up.' I'm going to demonstrate the 'classic sit-up' for you because it is pre-cisely the kind of exercise I want you to avoid. The starting position consists of lying flat on my back with my arms bent at the elbows and my hands clasped behind my head [fig. 12T]. Note that my legs are stretched flat on the floor and my feet are spread apart about eighteen inches.

"The exercise is performed by my sitting up and touching my elbows to

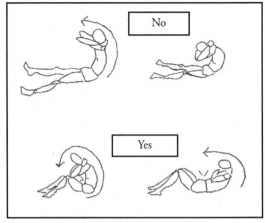

Fig 12T

my knees and then returning to the starting position. While there are many variations to this, they all suffer from the same defect: my straight legs put an enormous strain on my back. So, the first lesson we must learn is not to do this exercise with straight legs. Do them with bent knees and only with bent knees. This will take the strain off your back.

"You can do crunches with your hands clasped behind your head or with your arms folded in front of you. You can also do them by coming only halfway up and squeezing, or 'crunch-ing,' your abdominal muscles. I have often observed people doing them as fast as they can in an effort to do more and more reps. The actual num-ber of reps is far less important than the strength of the muscular contrac-tion. The important thing is to do them slowly and to try to squeeze your abs throughout the exercise. Hold it for a second or two at the halfway point before slowly returning to the starting position. Do as many as you can, then rest for a minute and try another set or two.

"Some fitness trainers insist that this type of exercise should include a variation where the elbows are alternatively made to touch the opposite knee. They believe that some of the abdominal muscles on the sides of our abdomens, known as the oblique muscles, are better exercised this way. However, there is little scientific evidence to support this contention.

"Sporting goods stores and other sales outlets have a number of different kinds of equipment that are designed to support your head and neck during these movements. Some others focus on roller-wheel mechanisms that can exercise your abs and some of the other muscles of your trunk at the same time. These are interesting and novel approaches that can serve to introduce some variety to your workout. But, enough about abs. Now let's talk a little about balance training.

Disturbances in balance

"Fractures are among the common causes of death in the elderly; and they are frequently the result of falls associated with balance problems. Disturbances in balance among older adults can result from a number of different conditions. To name a few of the more common causes: disturbances in the inner ear, visual disturbances, vascular disease involving the circulation to the brain, medications, and muscle weakness. Severe disturbances in balance or even mild disturbances of recent onset should be evaluated by your doctor.

Precautions against falling

"You can lower your risk of serious injury secondary to falls by following a few simple precautions.

1   First and foremost, begin to strengthen the muscles of your lower extremities and start a balance training program.

2   To make your bones stronger, take the medications, vitamins, and supplements (calcium and vitamin D) your doctor recommends.

3   Have your doctor or pharmacist review your other medications to determine if any might cause lightheadedness or drowsiness.

4   Identify risky habits. For example, don't walk with your hands in your pockets. If you lose your balance and start to fall, you might not be able to remove your hands fast enough to grab onto some support or break your fall.

5 Improve the safety of your surroundings by wearing non-slip shoes and placing non-slip mats and handrails in the bath or shower and on staircases.

6 Be certain that lighting is adequate throughout your household and that your carpeting is free of hazardous rumples.

7 Some of us older folks note rather marked dizziness with sudden changes in position. This is common with inner ear problems and also with sudden changes in blood pressure. Beware of quickly assuming the sitting position after an extended period of lying down or standing up suddenly after sitting for a long time. If you suffer from this type of balance disturbance, it's important to allow yourself time to stabilize when you change positions. If you're dizzy when you sit up from the reclining position, sit there and support yourself until you feel stable. Don't try to stand until you are stable. Then when you stand, support yourself with a hand on a chair or a tabletop until you feel stable enough to walk. Don't just start walking right away. These simple precautions might prevent you from falling and save you from the grief of a major bone fracture.

Balance training

"The leg and hip exercises we've demonstrated for strength training are extremely valuable in terms of improving balance. An increase in the strength of your lower body, in and of itself, will improve your balance. If you are doing your strength training at home, you can integrate balance training into these movements. But even if you do most of your strength training in the gym, you should add these movements purely for the purpose of enhancing your sense of balance.

"Let's revisit some exercises with our focus directed towards improving balance. These movements include the side leg raise, the hip flexion, the hip extension, the calf muscle exercise, and the chair stand. In most of these exercises, we've stressed the importance of holding onto the back of a chair for support. But you can improve your balance even more if you rely less on the support as your strength improves. As an example, in doing the side leg raise, gradually try to decrease your reliance on the chair for support. Hold on with two fingertips; and when you feel secure, try one fingertip.

"Hold the position for several seconds with each leg. As your balance improves, try letting go [fig. 12U] for a few seconds as long as support is nearby ('LOOK MA! No hands!'). Then you might even try it with your eyes closed for a few seconds. Repeat this with the hip flexion, hip extension movements, and the calf exercises. Try to gradually increase the time you can hold each position.

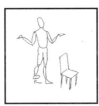

Fig 12U

Everyday activities

"Wherever you are, you can practice balance training by standing on one foot at a time for several seconds and then on the other foot. You can do this while talking on the phone [fig. 12V] or waiting in line at a store. When you rise from a chair, practice rising up without using your hands for assistance. The more frequently you try this, the better your balance might become.

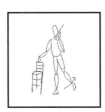

Fig 12V

Heel to toe walk

"There are also specific walking exercises that can be tried to improve your balance. One of the best is the 'heel to toe walk.' Place one foot progressively in front of the other, with the heel of one foot touching the toes of the other foot. This can be made even more difficult by using a line about three to four inches wide. A ten to twenty foot length of toilet paper on a smooth uncarpeted floor can be very useful here. Try to do a heel to toe walk without breaking or disrupting the paper.

Eye exercises

"Whether or not you can actually improve your vision with eye exercises is controversial. I believe there is real value to eye exercises that improve the motion of the eye, and also to some of the exercises that can help improve focusing and hand-eye coordination. Improved vision and eye-limb coordination can have a very positive effect on your balance. Clearly, there is no downside to doing these exercises. They're not even time-consuming. You can do them almost anytime and almost anywhere (but you have to take your glasses off). There are a number of variations to these exercises. Let's go over the three or four that I like the best.

- Clock rotation—Some research has shown that exercising the muscles responsible for moving the eyes, called the extra-ocular muscles, can improve vision. Sometimes, the improvement is immediately noticeable. Imagine that you are looking at the center of a large clock. Concentrate on the center of the clock and then move your eyes up to the twelve o'clock position, as far up as you can. Hold them and stretch them there for two or three seconds then return your eyes to the center position on the clock. Now repeat the same movement to one o'clock and then to two o'clock, and so on. Return to the starting position at the center of the imaginary clock each time. You can also try 'eye rolls.' Slowly roll and stretch your eyes out as far as possible around the clock, from the one o'clock position through to the twelve o'clock position and then back around the clock in the other direction.

- Far to near focus—Straining to focus our eyes by years of reading, working at a computer, or other kinds of near-point focusing changes the shape of our eyes. Over time, our eyes become rounder and fatter. This also occurs as a natural function of the aging process. To help prevent or possibly improve this defect, try the far to near focus exercise. Hold a pencil about six inches away and focus your eyes on any large object that is twenty to thirty feet away, like a telephone pole or a flagpole. Then quickly change your focus to the tip of the pencil. Repeatedly switch back and forth between the two

objects as quickly as you can, each time focusing as sharply as you can.

- Eye tracking—This is an exercise that requires you to keep your head still while following a fast-moving object with the movement of your eyes. Watching a tennis match or watching passing cars is a simple way to do this. Keep your head still and follow cars moving right to left across your field of vision by tracking them with your eyes. Then follow the cars moving from left to right across your field of vision. Keep your head as still as possible during this exercise. You can even try balancing a book on your head to assist you in keeping your head still.

- The Bungee Ball—It is a soft rubber ball about the size of a tennis ball that you can buy at many sporting goods stores. This is something all of us can enjoy. It's attached to an elasticized cord and has a wristband that prevents it from getting loose. Because of this, you can have fun with the bungee ball even if you're in a wheelchair or even if you only have use of one hand. Bungee balls can be used for exercising the extra-ocular muscles by eye tracking or for far to near focus. By swinging it far and near you can do some near to closer eye focusing exercises. By swinging it side to side you can do eye tracking exercises— but don't hypnotize yourself!

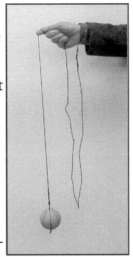

"In terms of improving hand-eye coordination, playing certain sports like tennis, racquetball, and ping-pong are wonderful. But for many of us who can't do this, the bungee ball is a good alternative. Because it's attached to your wrist and on a string, you can play catch with yourself without the concern of having to chase after a loose ball. You can throw it against a wall; you can throw it from hand to hand; or you can throw it up in the air and catch it with the same or opposite hand. It's a fun device that can really improve hand-eye coordination.

"Now that we're all so well-balanced, let's go into the aerobics room to work on endurance training."

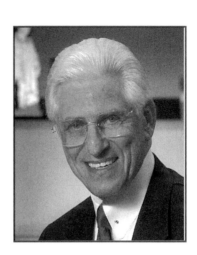

217

13

Your wind is the tender
To purchase insurance
That renders the splendor
Of greater endurance.

Aerobic Exercise and Maintaining Your Gain

The aerobics room was large. Stair climbers, treadmills, stationary bikes, rowing machines, and various other kinds of devices designed to exhaust the fittest of the fit were positioned along the walls. But the area was also designed to serve as an aerobics classroom and a lecture hall, as witnessed by the rows of folding chairs that occupied its central portion and the microphone/podium setup at the far end.

Oxygen debt

Zinney eased his way to the podium and, with microphone in hand, he began, "This is a slightly different world than the one you've been in. This is the world of aerobic exercise. You will recall our previous discussions on the difference between aerobic and anaerobic exercise. Aerobic exercise is also known as cardiopulmonary exercise or endurance training. This form of workout increases your heart rate for an extended period of time, thereby improving your cardiopulmonary conditioning. In large part, this is accomplished by carefully-paced exercise that avoids creating an *oxygen debt*. It's the *pay as you go* method of workout.

"Let me explain a little more by reminding you of the athlete who sprints a hundred yards in ten or eleven seconds. He will use about six liters of oxygen. But his maximum respiratory quotient, the most oxygen he can inhale, is about four liters a minute; yet, he used six liters in eleven seconds. So you see, he performed much of the sprint without oxygen— he owes his body oxygen. He created an oxygen debt. That's why you see him panting and gasping for breath after the race—he's paying back the oxygen debt.

Avoiding oxygen debt

"Aerobic exercise endeavors to avoid oxygen debt by pacing the exercise so that the oxygen you inhale is sufficient to fuel your muscles and clear the lactate as you workout. The exercises that best accomplish this are those that use our larger muscles, like our leg and back muscles. Brisk walking, jogging, and rowing are examples, as are aerobic classes. Marathon runners and long distance swimmers are probably among the most classic examples of advanced aerobic exercisers."

"From the pictures I've seen, these runners seem pretty short of breath at the end of the race. It seems that they created an oxygen debt," said Sheila.

"You're right, Sheila," Zinney responded. "Extended aerobic exercise eventually enters into an anaerobic phase where the oxygen required by the exercising muscles exceeds the ability of the cardiopulmonary system to deliver sufficient oxygen to the muscles. And so, oxygen debt develops. How quickly and to what extent this will occur in a given individual will depend upon that person's muscle and cardiopulmonary conditioning.

"There are three important factors that determine this efficiency. First, the condition of the lungs determines the ability to transfer inhaled oxygen into the blood stream. Second, the condition of the heart determines the ability of the heart to pump the oxygen-bearing blood to the muscles. And third, muscle conditioning determines the ability of the muscles to utilize the oxygen as it's delivered. So, you can see that heart disease, lung disease, and poor muscle conditioning can compromise your ability to do aerobics.

"Despite these conditions, almost anyone can dramatically improve their conditioning, their endurance, their zest, and their energy by a gradual and progressive approach to aerobics. For those of us who have been sedentary for a long time, our muscles may be weak or poorly conditioned so that we can't effectively indulge in aerobic exercise. In these situations, strength training is the first order of business. When our strength improves, we can go forward by adding endurance training to our program."

Is more better?

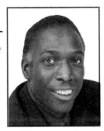

"Should we be striving to become marathon runners?" asked Leonard. "And also, what exactly did you mean when you said to gradually approach aerobic exercise?"

"Sure, Leonard. Gradual, gradual, and gradual are the important words to remember in your approach to cardiopulmonary conditioning. There is no rush. I want you to strive to gradually improve your performance. If you rush, you may hurt yourself and end up on the sidelines; and that setback may compromise all the gain you've accomplished.

"You've raised two important issues. I don't think we have to become marathon runners unless that's what you want to do. People who take to this, love it. It becomes a passion. With some exceptions, they don't generally compete with each other; they compete with themselves. They find real joy in attaining a level of superb cardiopulmonary fitness. This is 'fitness for fitness' as opposed to 'fitness for health.'

"While I do believe that each of us should attain a high level of fitness, there is a level of fitness above which there doesn't appear to be any additional health benefits. You see this high level of fitness, fitness for fitness, in competitive athletic endeavors such as in professional prizefighters, basketball players, competitive weightlifters, marathon runners, and the like. Sport injuries are so common in these athletes that attempting to get to that fitness level might, in some cases, be more of a health hazard than a health benefit. Achieving this extraordinary level of fitness should be motivated by the love of the sport as opposed to doing it for health benefits.

Target heart rate range

"Many experts believe that aerobic exercise should increase your heart rate to your 'target heart rate' range and maintain it at that level for twenty or thirty minutes three times a week. Doing this seems to produce as much cardiopulmonary health benefits as pushing yourself beyond that point, like becoming a competitive marathon runner. But using the target heart rate range as a guide to effective endurance training does not apply to everybody. And, again, it should be approached gradually."

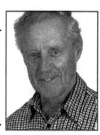

Craig asked, "So, how do you know your target heart rate? Isn't it different for everyone?"

"You're right. The so-called 'target heart rate' range or THR range varies with your age. Here's how to calculate what your THR should be. The magic starting number is 220. Subtract your age from 220 to determine your maximum heart rate. Then take 75 percent to 80 percent of that number to determine your THR. As an example, let's say you are sixty years old.

220 (the magic number) − 60 (your age) = 160 maximum heart rate

160 heart beats/minute = maximum heart rate (never exceed it)

Now take 80% of 160: .8 x 160 = 128 THR

"That's the THR—128 beats per minute. I don't think you should exceed it. You might view it as the *upper limit* of your target range. The *lower limit* might be about ten or twenty beats per minute less. To establish a reasonable range, subtract ten or twenty from your THR.

Therefore, your THR range = 108 to 128 beats per minute

"Your goal, if you're sixty years old, is to keep your heart beating between 108 and 128 beats per minute for 20 to 30 minutes during aerobic exercise and to do it three times a week.

"Count your pulse by using the index and middle fingers of one hand with gentle pressure to the outer part of the upturned wrist of the opposite forearm. Practice this now. Count the number of pulse beats for twenty seconds on your wristwatch and multiply by three. That gives you the number of times your heart is beating each minute. Do it frequently while you are exercising. If you want to go high tech, you can buy a device at some sporting goods stores that will measure your pulse and blood pressure. These gadgets fit on your wrist or on your finger. However, if you develop shortness of breath or if your heart is beating too fast, slow down or stop; and resume exercising at a slower pace.

"If, for example, while you're jogging, you feel you can't carry on a normal conversation with an imaginary person jogging next to you, then you are probably entering into an anaerobic stage of exercise. You're probably developing oxygen debt. This is a thought you should keep in mind with any of your aerobic endeavors whether it's bicycling, stair stepping, jogging, or brisk walking. This is a way of identifying shortness of breath—before it becomes overtly apparent. So as we said, slow down or stop and resume exercising at a slower pace. If you get chest pain, dizziness, or disturbing palpitations during exercise, stop and get it checked out by your physician.

"Please understand, it's not your goal to have your heart racing all the time, especially when you're at rest. As your conditioning improves, your heart rate at rest will actually get slower. That's because your heart has become more efficient, it can pump more blood with each beat. It's not at all unusual for a well-conditioned athlete to have a resting pulse rate between 50 and 65 beats per minute.

"You should be aware of some other features in using the THR range for establishing your cardiopulmonary conditioning. Don't expect to reach your THR range and maintain it for twenty minutes right away—unless you're already in pretty good shape. If you haven't been exercising, it will take time to condition your heart, your lungs, and your muscles so that they are able to perform at this level."

"How important is this THR stuff anyway?" asked Craig.

"It's not a must for good conditioning," Zinney answered. "There are those of us who may be taking a medication that prevents our heart rate from increasing. So, if you're taking medication, check with your doctor before starting a program that utilizes THR. Also, some of us older folks have an irregular heart rhythm or some other longstanding medical conditions that could prohibit our using this technique. Even though you don't need the THR range to improve your endurance, it's a good guide to cardiopulmonary conditioning.

Treadmill testing, peak exercise capacity, and metabolic equivalents [MET]

"If you want to get a more accurate determination of how fast your own heart should beat during exercise, have a treadmill test done by your physician. This could be of considerable importance if you haven't been exercising for awhile. Additionally, the treadmill evaluation can be used to assess your peak exercise capacity. The peak exercise capacity is measured in units called metabolic equivalents, or METs. Recent studies suggest that peak exercise capacity, as determined by a treadmill examination and adjusted for age, is probably the best predictor of mortality among men, when compared to other established risk factor for cardiovascular disease. If you score in the low range [< 4METs], your chances of having a serious cardiovascular event are four times higher than if you score in the high range [> 8 METs]. Some studies have shown that each 1-MET increase in peak exercise capacity confers a 12 percent improvement in survival from a cardiovascular problem. Moreover, your individual MET score can be used as a monitor to gauge your progress. So, as you gradually improve your exercise ability, you can improve your MET score, increase your longevity, and enhance your vitality.

How to start and progress

"Regardless of which form of aerobic exercise you choose, start slowly and progress gradually. Remember to always warm up and stretch before starting. You might begin by walking or jogging a quarter or a half of a mile, but progress gradually. If you haven't been exercising, you may have to start with as little as five minutes a day. That's ok. If that's your situation, try to gradually get up to ten minutes for each endurance session and then try to do two of these sessions a day. Then, build upon this progress until you can do twenty minutes at a time once a day. This is true whether your choice of exercise is

walking, using the treadmill, using a stationary bike, jogging, or whatever.

"When you feel the amount of exercise you're doing is easy, add a few minutes to the workout every ten to twenty days until you're doing thirty-minute endurance workouts. Then, when this is easy, quicken the pace or the difficulty of your exercise a little."

"You don't have to worry about me," said Sam. "I'm not gonna push too hard."

"Well," said Zinney, "you do have to push a little if you want to progress."

"I know. I know" said Sam. "I thought of a little ditty that might sum up how *I* feel:

> *"Listen up, Doc,*
> *I'm no croc,*
> *But when I huff and puff,*
> *I've had enough."*

"Well, you're right," said Zinney. "If you're huffing and puffing, you have had enough and you should slow down."

"Endurance is really important in cardiopulmonary conditioning," Leonard chimed in. "Remember, you and you alone are responsible for improving your endurance. You gotta be careful about making excuses for yourself. You have to push yourself a little. So:

*"Get off your duff
and strut your stuff,
'Cause you're the jock
that winds your clock!"*

"What clock are you talking about?" asked Sam.

"You know," Leonard responded, "the biological clock that Dr. Zinney told us about when we first started these meetings."

"Wow! You two are great. You should team up as rappers or something," said Zinney. "But let's get on with some other questions. I see Bertha has a question."

Frequency

"Yes, thank you, Dr. Zinney. I'd like to know how often us girls should be doing aerobics?"

"There's no gender issue here, Bertha. Some experts think you should be doing some form of exercise for thirty minutes every day. If you're able to do that, I think it's a good idea. But as I've said before, you should try to do endurance training three days a week, strength training at least two days a week, and stretching every day."

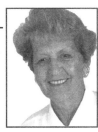

"Which of these aerobic exercises is the best?" asked Miriam. "You've talked about using the treadmill and walking, jogging, circuit training—which is best?"

"Miriam, there is no best. There's also swimming, running, brisk walking, stair stepping, martial arts, yoga and a host of other activities including some everyday chores that qualify as good endurance training. You can get an endurance workout mowing the lawn, raking leaves, or mopping the floor. But there is no best. Each of them has some advantages and some drawbacks, and each of you will find or develop your own preference.

Swimming and aquabatics

"Swimming is a great aerobic exercise that can also improve your strength. Exercising in the pool is often termed *aquabatics* or *aquaerobics*. For many, it's very enjoyable and refreshing; and because it's a low impact exercise, it's not likely to injure your joints. Equally important, because of the buoyancy provided by the water, excessive body weight doesn't compromise one's ability to workout. This can be of particular value to obese people. The buoyancy factor also assists in terms of stretching and resistance training.

"In terms of cardiopulmonary conditioning, however, most of us are not excellent swimmers. Our strokes and our kicks are less than perfect and our breathing technique is usually poor. As a result, many of us find ourselves gasping for breath before we've had a really good workout. But if you're a very good swimmer, swimming can be a wonderful way to combine aerobics with strength training and stretching. Even here, one of its advantages is also a disadvantage: swimming is a low impact exercise. While this decreases the chances of joint injury, it does little to prevent osteoporosis or increase bone mineral density. You need greater stress on your bones or a moderate amount of impact in your exercise program for this.

Stair stepping

"Stair stepping is another one we mentioned. More of us can indulge in stair stepping for aerobics than in swimming. You can actually climb up and down a flight of stairs or you can use a stair stepping machine. There are many variations in stair stepping machines including some that work your arms at the same time you're working your legs. You can get an excellent aerobic workout with this exercise in addition to some strength training for both your upper and lower body. But it's much more of an aerobic workout than a strength training activity. And here again, it's a low impact exercise that protects your joints but has little effect on improving bone density.

Walking and biking

"Now, let's talk a little about walking and bike riding. Most of us can participate in walking and some of us in biking as well. You can pick a safe and pleasant place to walk or bike and enjoy the sights while getting a nice workout; or you can use a treadmill or stationary bike in front of a TV screen.

"A brisk walk for forty-five to sixty minutes will burn about one hundred calories per mile. Casual walking, although a weight baring exercise, is not likely to produce enough impact to improve or maintain bone strength (see page 150). This is important to keep in mind if you do your walking at shopping malls. However, if you can't walk briskly, casual walking is far better exercise than no exercise as all.

"If you walk 3.5 miles in an hour, you're walking a mile every seventeen to eighteen minutes, a nice clip. Many of us can't do that to start. We may only be able to walk a quarter of a mile. That's about once around the block or once around the outside perimeter of a football field. Start slowly and gradually increase your distance and then increase your speed.

"If walking is your sport, try walking up a not-too-steep hill. You can push yourself a little, but not too far. If you get too short of breath or too fatigued, you should slow down or stop for a while. And when you finish your workout, you're not finished. You have to cool down with a little slow walking and stretching. Don't forget to stretch!

"Also, many treadmills have an adjustable incline so that you can increase the difficulty of the exercise as well as the speed. Some of the more sophisticated treadmill machines and stationary bikes also have pulse meters and calorie counters. This helps those of us who want to use the THR range to monitor pulse rate and caloric expenditure while we're working.

"Once again, low impact exercise like swimming, stair stepping and biking may not produce enough stress on your bones to enhance bone strength—unless you do them frequently and vigorously. Don't get me wrong, they are excellent endurance training activities. But if they are the only exercises you do, you might consider jogging in place for a minute or two after your workout. The impact provided by this might help to increase bone strength.

Jogging and jog-breaking

"Jogging and running are both high impact exercises. They're very popular and very good cardiopulmonary exercises that can have a significantly positive effect on bone mineral density. Their downside is the possibility of joint injury—especially to ankles, knees, hips, and low back as a result of the constant jarring. Here again, start slowly and progress slowly, particularly if you've been sedentary. An interesting way to get into this, if you have been sedentary, is to start with brisk walking. After you're comfortable doing this, try a jog-break— interrupt your walk every five minutes with ten or twenty seconds of jogging. After you've done this for a week or two, try jogging for thirty to sixty seconds every five minutes. As your conditioning improves, you can progressively increase the amount of jogging and decrease the amount of walking. Then, voila—you're jogging. And if you want to run, go faster. These are wonderful and highly addictive endeavors. But please remember that *gradual* is the important word.

Aerobics classes

"I heard somebody, there in the middle of the group mention aerobics classes. Here too we have an excellent form of both cardiopulmonary conditioning and stretching. Most of the better programs are divided into beginner, intermediate, and advanced aerobic classes. These classes are often a lot of fun. They stimulate energy and enthusiasm. They encourage a sense of social interaction and individual, as well as group, achievement. Despite this, many aerobic classes fail to address the specific needs of the individual participants. Each of us has a different level of fitness, especially in the beginner class. Those of us at a lower level are sometimes unwittingly seduced into trying to keep up with the group. It's our competitive nature. On one hand, this can be motivating; but on the other hand, it can be harmful. Some people might workout harder than they should and do some things they shouldn't—resulting in injury. Aerobics classes can be wonderful but be sure that your instructor is knowledgeable and attentive to your individual condition. If he or she is not, then find a different instructor.

Inter-relation of endurance and strength training

"Endurance training and strength training are not mutually exclusive—just the opposite. They are inter-related. They are kissing cousins. They're like the horse and carriage. If you have a marked decrease in muscle strength, you cannot perform endurance-training exercises effectively. As we've previously said, if this is your situation,

strength training is the first order of business for you. It's the most important thing you can do. Clearly, when you have improved your strength, your endurance will also have been improved. At this point, if you use some of the endurance training techniques we've discussed to further improve your endurance, your strength training program will also benefit. You'll be able to use more resistance and do more for longer. However, you can combine a strength training workout with an aerobic workout by circuit training.

Circuit training

"If you've been strength training and you're beginning to shape up, you can modify your strength training sessions so that you also get a good cardiopulmonary workout. This can be achieved by circuit training, by going from one resistance exercise to the next after just one set. Do this by decreasing the resistance, increasing the number of reps, and decreasing the rest periods between your circuit of exercises. Here's how to do it:

- Reduce the weight/resistance that you use in your usual workout by 50% or more for each resistance exercise.

- Do just one set of each resistance exercise; but increase the number of reps in each exercise, with this

228

lighter weight, from your usual eight or twelve reps to fifteen or even twenty-five reps.

- As you go from one resistance exercise to the next, decrease the rest periods between resistance exercises to thirty or even down to ten seconds.

- Continue to repeat the circuit until you've worked out for thirty minutes.

"As I've said, spending more time exercising your larger muscles, like the leg and back muscles, is likely to give you a better cardiopulmonary workout than working smaller muscles, like your biceps or triceps. So work more on the leg press, leg extension, leg curl, and back machines.

Interruptions

"If you have had to interrupt your workout schedule for a couple of weeks, resume your exercise program slowly. Don't expect to pick up where you left off right away. For the first week that you're back at it, start with half the resistance you usually use for strength training; and do half the amount endurance training you usually do. Then increase it to seventy-five percent for the second week. From there on, gradually increase your workouts to your prior level.

"You will get there. Don't panic. There's no rush. If for some reason, you lay off for two or three months, you may lose the gain you've achieved and you may have to start from scratch. Because of illness, this kind of layoff may be unavoidable, but don't let this happen voluntarily—stay with it. If, for whatever reason this does occur, think of how good you felt when you were fit and start again. Don't be disheartened.

Overwork

"Sometimes our muscles need more rest or recuperative time. This is particularly true among some older adults, but it can happen to anyone at any age. Often, but not always, this follows an unusually strenuous workout. In these cases, forty-eight hours may be insufficient for our muscles to repair and ready themselves for the next effort. When we try to work them out, we find that we perform less satisfactorily than we did on our prior workout. We get depressed and come to believe that we're regressing or failing to progress. Don't get down in the mouth about this. This too is normal. Give yourself a longer rest. Take seventy-two hours off and start again. If you still find yourself on a continuous down slope, or if you get dizziness, chest pain, or palpitations when you exercise, see your doctor for a checkup.

Maintaining the maintenance— the challenge for strength and endurance

"Well, now that you are all so wonderfully fit, how do you maintain this level of fitness? Let's take a look at what is likely to happen. If you've been sedentary, it's common to find significant improvement in your ability to workout and your fitness in just one month. Then, your improvement is likely to be more gradual and peak at the end of about eight to twelve weeks. Many of us will continue to progress, but it will probably be more gradual than the more dramatic improvement we achieved in the first twelve weeks. You might also note that some workouts and some weeks are better than others, or other times when your performance today is less than it was a week ago. This can be normal and doesn't necessarily mean that you're regressing. As we've said, there can be many reasons for this. You may have had a long layoff from working out because of illness or some other reason. You may have been working out too hard or too much and you haven't allowed sufficient time for your muscles to recuperate.

"By now, all of us recognize that in order to progress we need to gradually increase the resistance we use in strength training and gradually increase the intensity or the length of the exercise in endurance training. Now, in reality, building further and building more does have its limits. The ability to increase strength or endurance is not infinite—unless you're a Samson reincarnate. Your capacity to improve can be defined by your age, by your dedication to exercise, and by your genetic make up.

"But when you've achieved the strength and fitness level you desire, you want to maintain it. To do this for strength maintenance, most people establish a routine of doing a designated number of reps and sets with a designated resistance. We've discussed all this before [chapter 11 and chapter 12]. For cardiopulmonary conditioning, most of us will perform a specific endurance exercise a certain number of times each week at a specific level of intensity over a designated period of time. However, many have found that in using an exercise maintenance program that is consistently non-progressive, they actually enter a regressive stage. In other words, the maintenance program becomes increasingly more difficult to perform; and sometimes, they regress.

"The best way to avoid this is to challenge yourself on a regularly scheduled basis. For example, I've found it useful to challenge my routine once every ten to fourteen days by slightly increasing the weight or resistance I use for one set of each of the movements in my strength training exercises. Alternatively, you might try increasing the number of reps in a set or two once every two weeks. I also, try to slightly increase the difficulty or length of my usual endurance exercise once every ten days to two weeks. I think these small occasional challenges can help maintain the integrity of your maintenance program.

"Well, here we are again, my good friends. It's time to call it a night. For the next two weeks, our last two weeks together, we're moving back to the lecture hall in the community center. I know that we'll have record attendance next week because we have experts in our audience who might have commentary—we'll be discussing sexual activity in the older adult. See you then and have a good week."

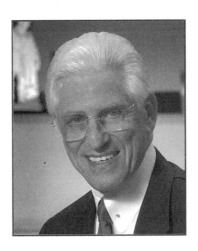

14

Sexual Activity in the Older Adult

Attention to your cleanliness
Can increase your lover's friendliness.
And if you carefully self-inspect,
You'll improve your self-respect.

A clear air of anxiety, coupled with excitement, was evident by the giggles and muffled laughter as people took their seats. Everyone knew that the subject for tonight's meeting could be spicy. Dr. Zinney wasted no time in getting the meeting started with, "Well, I can see from all the squirming going on out there that a lot of you are anticipating an exciting evening. So in the interest of preventing civil disobedience and satisfying His or Her Horniness's insatiable thirst for carnal knowledge, let's begin the discussion on sexual activity in the older adult. And also, let's talk a little about personal hygiene, appearance, and manners because they're related in so many ways."

Sex in the older adult

"For many of us older folks, sex actually becomes even more pleasurable. This might be because of a decrease in the pressures associated with meeting work-deadlines, keeping appointments, avoiding pregnancy, and the like. Even in nursing homes, romantic relationships develop that may culminate in sexual activity. Many compassionate attendants learn to look the other way. Some establishments even provide a comfortable surrounding for these events. Others prohibit them and even chastise the residents for these consensual interludes. This isn't to say that our sexual function remains unchanged as we age. But a better understanding of these changes and how to deal with them can help prevent the despair that deepens the pit of inactivity.

Frequency

"It should come as no surprise to most of you that there really is sex after forty. In fact, there's even sex after eighty. About 60 percent of men and women between the ages of forty to sixty years of age engage in some form of sexual activity about once a week. More than 25 percent of people seventy-five years of age and older also do it almost once a week. With advancing age and declining health, the frequency and type of sexual activity among couples varies progressively from once a week to three or four times a year to none at all. Under such circumstances loving relationships and cuddling, while always important, become even more important. Depression, chronic pain, de-fitness, lack of communication, hormonal changes, medications, belief systems, erectile dysfunction, and a host of other issues all combine to diminish libido and decrease sexual activity."

Craig leaned over and said to Sam, "This reminds of the story of these two old men. One was ninety-five and the other was ninety.

"The younger man asked the older man, 'Are you still doing it?'

"After a moment's consideration the older man responded, 'Of course I'm still doing it.'

"'Well, are you doing it once or twice?' asked the younger man.

"'Twice,' he responded.

"'Well, which do you like better—the first time or the second time?' asked the younger man.

"After a brief pause, the older man answered, 'I think I like the one in the Spring the best.'"

Zinney could tell from sporadic and scattered chuckles throughout the room that people were joking with each other. Confident that he had probably heard them all and fearful that airing them aloud might be offensive to some of the audience, he smiled and continued with the discussion.

Libido

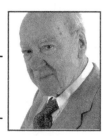

"What exactly is the libido?" asked someone in the audience.

"The term 'libido' simply refers to sexual desire, the desire to have sex. Libido, to some extent, varies with gender. For example, one study has shown that men think about sex on an average of once an hour and

234

women think about it less frequently—about two or three times a day. We have to be careful about how we interpret this stuff. This only suggests that it's on the minds of men more frequently throughout the day and not necessarily that women enjoy it less.

Intrinsic hormonal changes

"But what are the things that affect libido? And what could or should we do about them? To get a clear understanding of this, I like to discuss the issue from two standpoints: intrinsic and extrinsic factors. By intrinsic factors I am referring to hormonal changes. There can be no doubt that there is a decrease in sex hormones as we age. Postmenopausal women produce significantly less estrogen than their younger counterparts; and older men produce significantly less testosterone. In women, this can result in emotional changes that are associated with a decrease in libido, a decrease in energy, and a decrease in vaginal lubrication. In men, the decrease in testosterone may also be associated with a decrease in libido, de-fitness, and erectile dysfunction.

"Vaginal lubricants and, in selected cases, estrogen therapy can be very effective for some women. Less often, testosterone therapy can be partially effective in some of us guys. I say partially effective because the major impediments to sexual activity are, in most instances, not due to the intrinsic hormonal deficiencies but to a potpourri of extrinsic factors.

Extrinsic factors

Depression and medications "Chronic depression, medications, and the fear of failure loom high on the list for causing sexual difficulties. Couple this with the fact that many medications used to treat depression may adversely affect libido. In fact, many medications used to treat everything from ulcers to high blood pressure, can diminish the sexual appetite and some can even cause erectile dysfunction.

"If you're having trouble with your sexual appetite or your erection and you're taking medicine, ask your doctor about a possible cause and effect relationship. I'm sure you are all aware that excessive alcohol can also do this. So, if it's love you *choose*, don't over-*booze*.

Fear of failure "All you guys out there know what I mean when I talk about the fear of failure. Every man will, at one time or another, experience impotence and be unable to get an erection. This is normal. These occasional episodes may result from fatigue, worry, depression, or anxiety. These

intermittent episodes are not necessarily a sign of weakening sexual ability—they occur in almost everybody. However, sometimes the episode can be so traumatic that it creates a level of anxiety that perpetuates even more fear of failure. The important thing is to understand it for what it is. It's temporary; it's not abnormal; it's not a disease. You have to stop worrying and get on with your fun.

"A similar phenomenon can occur with the ladies. You may be used to having orgasms on a regular basis. Then one, two, or more times in a row this fails to happen. You become convinced it's over—you'll never have another orgasm. You're disappointed and perhaps even depressed. This can happen to any of you from time to time. It also can be the result of anxiety or worry or even illness. At other times, it's the result of a lack of communication between you and your lover or boredom with the lovemaking technique. If you're not satisfied, talk it out and try to work it out. Try different approaches or different positions. Discuss your fantasies with your partner. Under these circumstances, there's no substitute for candor. But the candor should be delivered with care to avoid hurt feelings. If this doesn't work, consider consulting a specialist in the field.

Chronic disease and chest pain "We all know that making love requires a significant amount of exertion—exertion that can cause a little shortness of breath, if you do it right. Chronic lung disease that compromises breathing can aggravate this situation to the extent that sexual activity becomes undesirable or even impossible. The same can be said for congestive heart failure and for unstable angina.

"Chest pain caused by the exertion of lovemaking can be frightening and make the very thought of sex undesirable and even dangerous. If you are so afflicted, it's important that you check with your doctor. He or she may be able to treat these problems so that sex can once again be enjoyable and safe.

De-fitness "De-fitness is a different issue. Some people are simply so out of shape or so obese that they don't have the physical endurance for sex. They convince themselves that they're no longer interested in it. Well, that's what we've been talking about these past several weeks—getting fit to win in the second half. That means exercising, eating right, and quitting smoking. Getting fit will not only make you *look* sexier, it will make you *be* sexier. You'll have more stamina, more desire, more zest for life, and more fun—for you and your partner. The stretching exercises you've learned are very important. If you're more flexible, you will have greater ease of motion. In other words, if you improve your *flexibility*, you may increase your *sex ability*.

Painful sex "Painful sex, in both males and females, should be divided into two categories. One is pain in the genital area during intercourse and the other is pain outside the genital area. It's important to distinguish between the two. People with arthritis, low back pain, and chronic abdominal discomfort are often limited in many of their activities, including sex. In those with chronic arthritis or low back discomfort, simply taking their anti-inflammatory medication prior to making love will often permit a more enjoyable experience. Also, it may help to try positions other than the missionary position for comfort as well as for variety and enjoyment. We'll talk about that a little bit later.

"Then there's discomfort in the genital area when having sex. While, both men and women can experience pain in the genital area during sexual intercourse, it's somewhat more common among women and is often the result of inadequate vaginal lubrication. Some men just don't allow

enough time for their partner to be sufficiently aroused or don't do enough gentle petting before attempting penile insertion.

"Listen up, guys—that can hurt your partner. So take your time and be gentle. Some gentle sexual petting can do a lot to help with vaginal lubrication and vaginal elasticity. This can make it a much more enjoyable experience for the both of you. As I said, there's no doubt that natural vaginal lubrication can decrease with advancing age; but this is easily remedied with the use of vaginal lubricants applied before sex. You can find them in any drugstore, or ask your doctor for a recommendation.

"You guys can also experience discomfort in the genital area when having sex. Usually this is the result of an irritation or an infection in this region. An inflammation of the urinary bladder or the urethra, the tube that leads outward from the bladder through the shaft of your penis, can cause discomfort during sex or while you're passing urine. This kind of inflammation can happen in both men and women. Pain on ejaculation can be experienced as a result of an inflammation of the prostate gland or the seminal vesicles, the pouches that hold and empty your semen [fig. 14A]. Most often the cause of these conditions can be quickly diagnosed and cured with a trip to your doctor. So if you want that *lay,* don't de*lay.*"

Prostatitis and the prostate gland

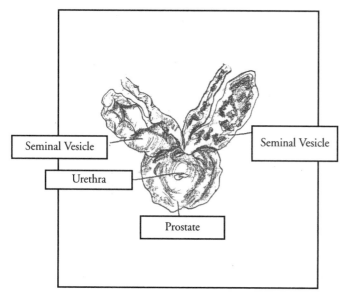

Fig 14A

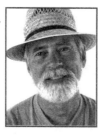

"Well, wait a minute, Doc. I'm not sure I understand exactly what the prostate gland is or does," said John. "And, I hear a lot about enlargement of the prostate. What about that?"

"Okay. Let's start by talking a little about the gland itself," replied Zinney. "The prostate gland is normally about the size of a chestnut, but it can enlarge to the size of a big orange. It surrounds the first inch or two of the urethra [fig.

14A] and is composed of glandular material and strands of muscle. Some of the muscle fibers that surround the first inch of the urethra blend with the muscle fibers of the bladder. While it doesn't produce any hormones, the glandular elements of the prostate secrete a fluid that, together with the fluid of the seminal vesicles, is added to the sperm during ejaculation. Being situated in the front of the rectum, most of the back side of the gland can be easily felt during a rectal examination.

Benign Prostatic Hyperplasia (BPH)

"A condition called Benign Prostatic Hyperplasia, or BPH, is the most common cause of prostate gland enlargement. The term hyperplasia is used to indicate an increase in the number of cells. This increase can cause anything from a mild to a massive enlargement of the gland. The enlarged gland, along with spasticity of the prostatic musculature, encroaches on the urethra and impedes the flow of urine.

"This can give you a myriad of unpleasant symptoms. The obstruction of urinary flow results in incomplete evacuation of the bladder causing urinary frequency throughout the day and it may even disturb your sleep with the need to void several times during the night. You might also experience any or all of the following symptoms: difficulty in starting urination, diminished size and force of the urinary stream, post urinary dribbling, or even an overflow dribbling incontinence. Excruciating urinary urgency and bladder distension may be experienced, especially if *acute urinary retention* occurs.

"On rare occasions, this can happen without warning and in others it is precipitated by repeatedly denying the urge to void or taking some seemingly innocent medications that can aggravate urinary retention, such as bowel relaxants (anticholinergics), decongestants, and antihistamines. When total obstruction to urinary flow occurs, as in acute urinary retention, emergency measures in the form of catheterization or surgery may be necessary. To make matters worse, the retention of urine can predispose you to recurrent urinary tract infections and damage your urinary bladder. The progressive stretching of the bladder wall can weaken the wall and result in the formation of pockets or out-pouchings called bladder diverticuli."

The cause of BPH

"What causes all this, and why does it happen?" asked Craig.

"The reason this happens and increases in frequency with advancing age is

not clear—it's a bit of a puzzle. Microscopic studies on prostate gland tissue have shown that hyperplasia increases in frequency from eight percent of men aged 31 to 40 years, to fifty percent of men 51 to 60 years, to more than eighty percent of men who are older than eighty years of age.

"Here's the puzzle: We know that testosterone increases the growth of the prostate, and we know that testosterone production decreases with advancing age. Therefore, we would expect the prostate gland to decrease in size with advancing age; but, that's not what happens. Some investigators theorize that the threshold of prostatic tissue for the action of testosterone is lowered as age advances to an extent that more than compensates for the diminished production of testosterone. Others postulate that the conversion of testosterone to DHT (dihydrotestosterone), the active form of the hormone responsible for prostatic growth, is increased. Still others speculate that prostatic hyperplasia results from an imbalance between estrogen and testosterone that occurs with aging. Simply stated, it happens; and we just don't know why. Hopefully, ongoing research will give us some answers in the near future.

Treatments and precautions

"The treatment your doctor will recommend will, in large part, be determined by the severity of your symptoms, the size of your gland, your age, and the presence or absence of other complicating diseases. With less than severe symptoms and with mild to moderate enlargement of the gland, you will probably do very well with medical therapy.

"If you experience a sudden increase in urgency or frequency, or if you develop burning on urination or blood in your urine, your condition is most likely complicated by a urinary tract infection (UTI). See your doctor. He or she may recommend a urine culture and prescribe antibiotics. I would also suggest some common-sense precautionary measures that can reduce some of the distress associated with BPH.

"You can decrease urinary frequency by avoiding those things that might promote excessive urination like alcohol, or beverages containing caffeine. Surprisingly, many soft drinks have significant amounts of caffeine, so you have to read labels carefully. You might also save yourself a few wakeup calls if you avoid drinking beverages near bedtime.

"Many of my patients have described horror stories of being trapped in traffic jams when seized by a painful and almost undeniable need to urinate, and some have. Try to anticipate this, or similar problems, and make it a habit to urinate before leaving your home or place of business. Certain medications can aggravate the symptoms or even precipitate acute urinary retention in patients with BPH (anticholinergics, decongestants, antihistamines, etc.). I've known patients who were catapulted to the emergency room after taking a seemingly harmless cold remedy that contained a decongestant or antihistamine. However, some of the newer antihistamine drugs have a much lesser likelihood of causing this. So please, check with your doctor. Before leaving the subject, there's another bit of advice I'd like to give all of you fastidious gentlemen.
It goes like this:

> "Before you zip,
> please be hip.
> Shake your tip
> to shed that drip.
> If you close your fly
> before you dry,
> You'll be a sticky guy
> with an icky thigh.

Medications that can help "When the prostate gland isn't too large, disturbing symptoms and progressive damage to the urinary bladder can often be controlled with the use of medications called *alpha-adrenegic blockers* such as Hytrin, Cardura, or Flomax. These medications can relax the musculature of the prostate and allow for an easier egress of urine out of the bladder. In other words, they help open the gate that's guarded by the spastic musculature of the prostate gland around the first inch or two of the urethra. While they're all effective, I've seen the best results, with less side effects, in patients using Flomax.

"Another kind of medication called Proscar has been effective in decreasing the symptoms of BPH by arresting the growth or even reducing the size of the prostate. It works by blocking the conversion of testosterone to dihydrotestosterone (DHT). Some studies have suggested that it adversely effects sexual function—libido, potency, and the size of the ejaculate. Others have shown that these effects are no more frequent than they are with placebos. Unlike the *alpha-blockers,* Proscar takes time to work. You have to be patient. It is also important to note that this medication can artificially lower blood PSA determinations rendering a very valuable screening test for prostate cancer useless. "Some

European studies have suggested that the herb, saw palmetto, which is extracted from the saw palmetto berry, can produce results similar to Proscar. In my experience, this herb does seem to relieve symptoms associated with a large prostate in some patients. While I know of no evidence that it actually decreases the size of the prostate, I believe it to be safe and worth a try. You can buy it in most drugstores without a prescription.

Surgical options "In cases where the prostate has achieved massive enlargement, surgical removal of the prostate may be necessary. Concern regarding the development of sexual impotency following prostate surgery has struck fear into the hearts of many men. While these concerns are founded in reality, they are often exaggerated. Improved techniques have significantly reduced the frequency of this complication. Depending on the size of the gland and the type of surgery required, the incidence of this complication varies from five percent to less than twenty percent.

"Advanced enlargement usually requires open surgery; but in some cases, the removal of the gland can be accomplished with the use of small scopes inserted through the lower abdomen (laparoscopic prostatectomy). In most cases, if the gland is not massively enlarged, obstructing prostatic tissue can be removed with a small scope through the urethra.

"This lesser form of surgery is known as transurethral resection of the prostate (TURP). The majority of patients who require surgery can be effectively treated with a TURP. Recently, transurethral electrovaporization of the prostrate (TEVP) has grown in popularity. It consists of vaporizing the obstructing tissue with an electric current. While it does require hospitalization and spinal or general anesthesia, it appears to be associated with fewer complications and shorter hospital stays than a TURP.

"Similarly destructive procedures that can be done as an outpatient with local anesthesia are becoming popular. Some examples are High Intensity Ultrasound, Transurethral Microwave, and Transurethral Needle Ablation. However, the newest kid on the block is Water Induced Thermotherapy (WIT). In selected cases, it has shown very promising results with minimal discomfort and no reports of sexual dysfunction. Keep in mind that a urinary catheter is required for a few days after all of these surgical techniques. Each of these procedures has a cadre of enthusiastic physician advocates. For this reason, it's important to know that one shoe does not fit all feet. If

you need this kind of relief, be sure you have an experienced urological surgeon to help you decide which procedure is best for your case."

Sam leaned over and whispered to Craig. "I can't help thinking of these two old guys talking in the doctor's waiting room. The 85 year old told the 95 year old, 'I'm here to see the doctor because every day at 7 in the morning I have trouble making water. I stand by the toilet and squeeze and maybe I make a drop of urine. Then, at 8, I sit and grunt on the toilet and maybe make only a pebble of a bowel movement.' The 95 year old then responded, 'I don't have these problems. At 7 I make a bucket of urine and at 8 I make a big healthy bowel movement. The only problem is, I can't get out of bed until 9.'"

The normal erection and erectile dysfunction

John commented, "Zinney, you've mentioned erectile dysfunction several times. I'm sure that means difficulty in getting an erection. Can you tell us more about it now? What causes it and what can be done about it?"

"A very important question, John. Now is as good a time as any to talk about it. Erectile dysfunction is also referred to as 'ED.' It means an inability to achieve or maintain an erection of sufficient quality to have sexual intercourse. To have a better understanding of ED, it's probably a good idea to first review a little about the anatomy of the penis and the normal mechanism of erection.

"Basically, an erection occurs when the penis becomes filled with blood. The engorgement and trapping of blood in the penis is what causes the penis to enlarge, elongate, and stiffen. But this famous event involves a series of very complex reactions. Let me explain. In this slide, we see a cross section [fig. 14B] and a longitudinal section [fig. 14C] of the penis.

"As you can see, the main bulk of the penis is made up of two sponge-like structures known as the *corpus cavernosum* and the *corpus spongiosum*. It isn't important to remember these names if you don't want to.

"There are tiny nerves and muscle fibers in the tissue that makes up the sponge, between and around the spaces (sinusoids). When the penis is in its normal resting state, these little muscle fibers are contracted [fig. 14D].

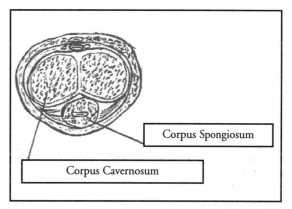

Fig 14B

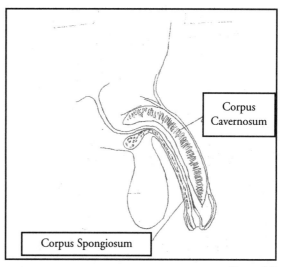

Fig 14C

"Uh oh. I can see a little question mark on some of your faces. But that's right—the little muscle fibers are in a contracted state when the penis is in the resting state. When these tiny muscle fibers relax, the sinusoids or spaces become more expandable, thus more able to receive more blood [fig. 14D].

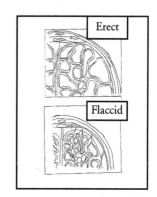

Fig 14D

243

"So you see, an erection is a complex series of events. Bloodflow to the penis increases from emotional, visual, or tactile stimulation. Messages transmitted by hormones and nerves signal the increase in bloodflow and signal the muscles in the sponge to relax. This allows blood to fill and expand the sinusoids, or spaces in the spongy tissue. As the sinusoids expand and enlarge, the veins, the channels that drain the sinusoids, are compressed. This traps the blood in the sponge-like structures of the penis and Voila!—an erection or hard-on, a boner, or woody.

"There's one important aspect that I didn't mention—*neurotransmitters.* You remember we mentioned them several weeks back when we talked about brain function [chapter 3]—we talked about serotonin and other chemicals released by nerve endings that assist in transmitting messages from one nerve to another or from a nerve to a muscle telling it what to do. Probably, the most important neurotransmitter in the mechanism of erection is *nitric oxide.* The release of this neurotransmitter triggers a series of events that causes the muscle in the sponge-like structures to relax. And as I said, the relaxation of these muscles allows the sinusoids to open up and fill with more blood.

"After Mt. Vesuvius erupts or fatigues, i.e. after ejaculation, the neurotransmitters are turned off and those muscles in the sponge-like structures contract into their normal resting state. This opens the veins, allowing the blood to be drained from the penis; and the erection fades. The penis returns to its inactive state. While now just 'a *softy,*' it's still proud and *lofty.*

The causes of ED in aging

"While there are many causes for ED, for the purpose of our discussion, we will focus our attention on those most relevant to the aging process. It's usual for sexual function to decrease with advancing age. We might note that it takes a longer period of sexual stimulation to produce an erection, that our erections are less firm and they don't last as long. We might also note that the period of time between our ability to get erections lengthens and that our penis is less sensitive to touch and other forms of stimulation. And we might even note that we just can't get an erection that works. But why?

"Sometimes the cause is purely physical. Sometimes it's because of psychological problems, such as anxiety or depression. Sometimes it's the result of the *fear of failure* factor previously discussed. Often, it's a combination of both the physical and the psychological.

"As you know from our discussion, an erection is the result of the penis becoming engorged with blood. Anything that decreases bloodflow to the penis or decreases its ability to fill, such as arteriosclerosis, can decrease penile engorgement and hamper the ability of the penis to become rigid. Cigarette smokers and people with diabetes are at particularly high risk for this. Scientists also suspect that, as we age, there is an increase in the tone of the muscle fibers in the spongy tissue of the penis. This could make it more difficult for the spaces (sinusoids) in this spongy tissue to receive blood. A decrease in testosterone production, diminished sensitivity of the nerves to the penis, and a decrease in neurotransmitters also develops with aging. If that's not enough, we have to appreciate that people are subject to a number of chronic diseases as they get older. As previously mentioned, many of the medications used to treat these conditions may have an adverse effect on producing an erection.

Treatment of ED

"Well, if you have ED, what should you do about it? The first thing you should do is see your doctor. He or she may make simple changes in your medication that will make all the difference in the world. In other instances, your doctor might recommend certain tests to identify the cause or causes of your ED. Psychotherapy and treatment by sex therapists have sometimes been helpful. Having said that, let me discuss some of the treatments that have been used over the years.

Surgical techniques

"In the early 1970s, penile prostheses were in favor. This consisted of the surgical insertion, into the penis, of a device that would keep the penis firm for performing intercourse. Improvement in these devices soon followed so that the penis could be pumped up or decompressed when desired. Among the disadvantages of this procedure, were those of infection, malfunctions, and the very fact that a surgical implantation was required. Still, many men and their spouses, in the absence of a better solution, opted to have the operation and many are still enjoying the results.

"In the next decade, surgical procedures to improve bloodflow to the penis became popular. Patients were studied to determine if there was a significant obstruction to the main artery to the penis. If there was, the obstruction was surgically remedied. This worked for some patients, but not for others; because as we discussed earlier, the cause of ED in our aging member is usually multi-factorial. Correcting the circulatory problem in the main artery did not necessarily improve bloodflow through the smaller branches nor did it address any of the other causes of ED.

Prostaglandins

"Let me introduce you to another substance called Prostaglandins. These are often called nature's protective substances. They are made naturally at several different locations in our body and it was known for quite some time that they play an important role in the process of erection. But to use them for the treatment of ED, they have to be administered either by a small needle injection directly into the side of the penis or by putting the medication into the urethra of the penis. The urethra, of course, is the channel or tube in the penis that transports our urine and ejaculations to the outside world. When patients are carefully instructed in the self-administration of these agents, this form of treatment proved highly successful for many.

"However, there are some important drawbacks. To mention a few: the inconvenience and discomfort of administration, urethral pain, and priapism. Before you ask the question, let me tell about priapism. Priapism is a painful and persistent erection. It can

have serious consequences and may require emergency treatment. Fortunately, it is uncommon."

Testosterone

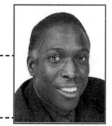

"What about testosterone injections?" asked Leonard.

"Generally speaking, I don't tout it much for most cases of ED in older men. While it is useful when there's a marked deficiency in testosterone, it can have long- and short-term side effects. Testosterone injections have great activity during the first week after injection and decrease thereafter. This can result in a roller-coaster effect characterized by jubilance, excitement, and even aggressiveness followed by fatigue, lassitude, and sometimes, severe depression.

"Oral testosterone treatment, in pill form, has been a problem because the only kind available in this country has been methyl testosterone. This form of testosterone has been associated with severe liver disease. However, more recently developed preparations of *testosterone undecanoate* are demonstrating good results with lesser hazards. The jury is still out on these and a number of other new preparations that are in the pipeline.

246

"More recently-developed testosterone skin patches have a much smoother effect than injection therapy. These patches can raise testosterone levels to normal in more than 90 percent of men. Sometimes they cause annoying skin irritations; but the even newer gel-type preparations appear to have substantially solved this problem. The gel preparations also seem to have a very positive effect on bone mineral density.

"My major concern with testosterone replacement therapy is in regard to its long-term effects on the prostate gland and the cardiovascular system. Testosterone may increase the growth of the prostate gland—a problem that should concern some of us older guys. Enlargement of the prostate gland can cause obstruction of the neck of the urinary bladder, which may require remedial surgery.

"The effect that testosterone can have on prostate cancer is an even greater concern. It could make it grow faster. Certainly, anyone with this form of cancer must avoid testosterone. And suppose some of us don't know if we have prostate cancer? Suppose we are walking around with undiagnosed prostate cancer, a prostate cancer with negative blood tests that might otherwise be so slow-growing that it doesn't threaten our lives? Should we nourish and encourage the growth of this can-

cer with testosterone? I think not! So you see, caution must be exercised in using this stuff. It's really important to have regular examinations of the prostate gland—both rectal exams and blood tests.

"Testosterone can also raise serum lipids, which promote the development of atherosclerosis and coronary artery disease. So if you're going to take this stuff, you should have your serum lipid levels checked at regular intervals.

Other medications

"A host of medications, such as *yohimbine, phentolamine, apomorphine, papaverine,* and *trazadone,* have been recommended for the treatment of ED all with some small degree of success and most with some undesirable side effects. Again, you don't have to remember the names. But none of these have had the impact and success of *Sildenafil*—otherwise known as *Viagra.* Now this stuff really works for most cases of ED and has very little downside. You remember the neurotransmitter we talked about earlier called nitric oxide. Through a complex series of reactions, Viagra causes an increase in the concentration of nitric oxide in the penis. This relaxes the smooth muscles in the sponge of the penis and allows the sinusoids to accept more blood and become more turgid. There you have it: *correction of erection without injection*. It's a pill.

"Viagra takes about an hour to start working; but after you take it, the medicine is usually effective for a period of four to five hours. Gentle sexual stimulation will most often produce a good erection. The usually mild side effects are those of nasal congestion, heartburn, headache, and flushing. For the most part, they are infrequent and transient. Rare cardiac problems have been reported; and for this reason, it's important for your doctor to determine if Viagra is right for you. Certain heart medications and blood pressure medicines represent an important contraindication to Viagra therapy. So please, don't just get the stuff from some Internet or black market source. Be smart and check with your doctor."

"Does Viagra have any effect on libido?" asked John.

"Most studies have shown that Viagra had little direct effect on libido," Zinney responded. "But it can have an indirect effect. If you're able to achieve an erection and enjoy sex, then your libido, your desire to have more sex, is likely to be increased."

"It seems that you really have to plan your sex if you have to wait an hour for it to start working. It takes the spontaneity out of it, doesn't it?" said Bertha.

"Yeah," John quipped. "It's sort of like going to an *amusement park*—a one hour wait for a three minute ride."

"Ha, ha! To some extent that might be true," answered Zinney. "But on the other hand, there's nothing wrong with a little planning for a really good time. Moreover, I'm sure that faster and longer acting versions of similar drugs are being developed—perhaps in the form of a sublingual version or nasal spray kind of product."

Hormone replacement therapy and sexuality in women

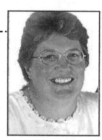

"What about hormone replacement treatment, Doc? Will that really improve our sexuality?" asked Bertha.

"As we discussed some weeks ago, estrogen replacement therapy by pill or by patches has many advantages in regard to sexuality but also, as we previously discussed, it has some disadvantages. Surely, estrogen appears to improve vaginal lubrication, libido, and skin texture, and combat insomnia in postmenopausal women. To some women, the ability of estrogen to alleviate hot flashes or night sweats and help to prevent osteoporosis is even more important. On the flip side, recent studies on women taking estrogen and progesterone (HRT) have yielded disturbing results. An increase in the frequency of breast cancer, uterine cancer, ovarian cancer, strokes, and heart attacks has been suggested. While the results of the study focused on women taking combination therapy (HTR), continued evaluation of women taking estrogen alone is part of an ongoing branch of this investigation. Fearing the results may be similar, I am inclined to wait for the verdict before endorsing estrogen replacement therapy across the board. Soy products and other plant estrogens as well as some herbs like black cohosh may provide some of the benefits of estrogen replacement therapy without its attendant risks. As an interesting aside, the addition of testosterone patches for some women who are also taking estrogen replacement therapy has recently been shown to increase their libido and their sense of well-being.

"You may not realize that testosterone is naturally present in gals—not just the guys. The ovaries are an important source of testosterone in the female. When they're removed by surgery, the testosterone level drops. This was demonstrated by a recent study on a select group of women who had a hys-terectomy and who had their ovaries removed. I'm not suggesting that any of you gals go out and start taking testosterone. You may start growing beards! There's a lot yet to be learned about the short- and long-term effects of testosterone replacement therapy in females.

Romance

"Now I'd like to spend some serious time discussing the idea of romance with all of you. I'm not talking about reciting poetry, although sometimes that could be a very good idea too. Many of you folks know the wisdom of remembering birthdays and anniversaries with a little gift of flowers or cologne. This is all very important. It can even be a good idea, once in awhile, to buy some cute or sexy lingerie. Whether the man buys it for his wife or the wife buys it herself, believe me, it can add a little spice to your life."

John tilted a little towards Leonard and said, "I got a good one about lingerie I just gotta tell you. It's about this very elderly couple. She went out and bought some new nighties and decided to try them on for her husband. So she went in the bathroom and came out wearing a sexy red one and asked, 'How do you think this looks, honey?'

"The old man squinted and said, 'Well, it fits real good but I don't much like the color.'

"So, she tried on a blue one and then a purple one; and each time he squinted and gave the same response, 'It fits real good but I don't much like the color.'

"Frustrated, she then came out naked and said 'How do you like this one, dear?'

"Once again the old man squinted and said 'Now I really like that color, but it sure needs an ironing.'"

"Ha! Ha! I don't think I'll share that one with my wife," said Leonard.

Demeanor and communication

"But what I want to talk about is, in my opinion, even more important than lingerie," continued Zinney. "I'm going to talk about some of the other features that made your courtship successful and contributed to the fun of your youth. These are features that some of us forget or take for granted as we get a little older or that we mistakenly believe aren't as important as they were when we were younger. I'm talking about your approach to your partner, your communication techniques, your manners, and your appearance—you know, your state of cleanliness and even your odor. All of this can go a long way in influencing the pleasure of your relationship.

"Many of you guys think that when you're ready, your partner is also ready. Not so, my good friends. The sword of Alexander the Great, your lonely erection, is not the equivalent of the bugle sounding the charge of the Light Brigade. Be patient. Don't scare your partner! Indulge in a little kissing and petting before thrusting yourself upon her like the alpha gorilla we men envision ourselves to be at that moment.

"Develop a form of communication, either verbal or physical, that both of you recognize and can respond to. Your partner may not be feeling well or for some other reason be unable to enjoy sex at that time. Both of you have to learn to accept that without getting angry. If this is an ongoing event, wherein the two of you can't get your timing right, then a candid discussion regarding the issue should be arranged. But it shouldn't be an argument. It shouldn't be a blaming session. It should be a gentle and constructive effort on the part of both partners. Most problems have solutions and both of you must participate in developing them."

John Kinder was sitting behind Craig and Sam and leaned over to say, "I gotta tell you this one about communication." The two listeners pertly positioned their ears in his direction as John proceeded.

"This guy says to his wife, 'Listen honey, when I want to have sex I'll reach over and stroke your left breast three times. And when you want sex, you reach under and stroke me three times.'

"His wife says 'But honey, what if I don't wanna have sex?'

"So the guy says 'Well, if you don't want sex then reach under and stroke me fifty times.' Ha, ha! Good one, huh?" chuckled John.

Personal hygiene

Zinney continued while smiling at Sam and Craig as they attempted to muffle their laughter, "Personal hygiene is important from a health standpoint apart from its influence on sexuality. But since we're discussing things that influence sexual activity, this seems like a good time to get into it. For most of you here tonight, this isn't applicable. Most of you appreciate the importance of cleanliness; but some of us become lax as we get older and place less importance on it than we should. This is often because we don't care about ourselves as much as we should. We lose our sense of importance and our self-esteem; or in other instances, we're just down-right lazy.

"Let's be frank! Some of us simply don't bathe as frequently as we should for whatever reasons. Dirt represents a real health hazard; and esthetically, nothing can turn your partner off more quickly than shmutz and stink. I remember as a kid, living in the cold northeast we were told that you didn't have to bathe every day because it dried out your skin. That's bull! Bathe or shower every day; and wear clean socks and underwear every day. A good moisturizing body lotion can be used daily to keep your skin from drying out.

"Remember, you can't smell yourself; so don't bother sniffing your armpit to determine whether or not you need to bathe or shower. Trust me, if you don't clean yourself, you're gonna stink. You won't know it but everybody else will. Your olfactory senses, the nerve endings in your nose that detect odors, quickly accommodate to odor. As an example, when you put on some cologne or perfume, in a very short while you can't notice it. But others can smell it.

"Also, as we age, our sense of smell isn't as sharp as it was when we were younger. That's why some ladies put on entirely too much perfume.

Sometimes older women and some men put so much of the stuff on that they literally reek. Be aware, my friends, our sense of smell ain't what it used to be—so don't go too heavy with cologne or perfume.

"Some older adults don't bathe or shower because of the fear of slipping or falling. In many cases, this is a reasonable concern. It can often be dealt with by making the bath or shower safer with rails, seats, and slip-retardant mats or tiles. Another alternative, that many couples find pleasantly effective, is to use the buddy system for bathing or showering—help each other wash and protect each other from falling.

Toilet hygiene

"In addition to bathing, there is the special issue of toilet hygiene. There are two ends to be tended to—brushing your teeth and cleaning yourself after a bowel movement.

"Sour breath is a big industry. There are hundreds of breath mints and remedies sold in stores and over hot lines. Superb marketing has attempted to produce mass paranoia. These marketing techniques are geared to convince the public that everybody needs these things because everybody has bad breath. To some extent, that's true. Everybody at one time or anoth-

er does have foul-smelling breath. And you can't really smell your own breath no matter how hard you try or whatever hand-cupping techniques you employ. Remember—you can't smell yourself. No doubt these breath mints and chewing gums can be refreshing from time to time. So if you enjoy them, have at it. But the important thing is to have a clean mouth, healthy teeth, and healthy gums. This is best accomplished by flossing and brushing your teeth after each meal, the most important path to clean breath. I know it's not always convenient, but certainly most of us can do this at least twice a day. Breath mints are okay, but they're not a substitute for good oral hygiene."

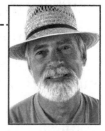

"What about those of us who have dentures?" asked John. "Sometimes they really smell bad."

"Dentures can cause a bad breath problem," Zinney responded. "Usually this can be well-controlled with proper cleaning of the dentures and using mouthwash.

Perianal cleansing

"On an even more delicate subject, some of us, as we age, aren't as careful as we should be after a bowel move-

252

ment. Some people just don't clean themselves. What could be more of a turn-off than residual fecal material between the cracks of a person's butt? You have to clean yourself carefully and thoroughly. This doesn't mean that you should scrub yourself raw. The skin around the perianal area is tender and should be treated tenderly. Vigorous scrubbing can irritate the skin and set it up for an infection. A good technique is to gently swab the area with wet toilet paper until it is clean and then blot it with dry toilet paper. I appreciate that some of us may have difficulty reaching back there because of physical limitations. In these cases, cleansing might be easier if you use some of those pre-moistened anal wipes. You can buy them at almost any drugstore.

Gaseousness

"Another delicate subject is intestinal gas. Everyone has intestinal gas and all of us have excessive intestinal gas from time to time. In some of us, it's more of a problem than it is in others. Occasionally, this causes us to burp or break wind—a very understandable situation. Most partners develop an understanding of the other partner's distress; and in this regard, they accommodate to each other's need to seek relief.

"However, some people unnecessarily expel gas at inappropriate times. To hear some of my patients tell it, their bed has become a *farting field*. Their spouses actually wait to get into bed before erupting. Sometimes they're silent and full of odiferous surprises; and at other times, they're a symphony of broken trumpets. The farters come to believe that their partners are used to it; so it doesn't matter. In some cases that's true. But in others, it has a very negative conscious or even unconscious effect on the romance of your bed—where you sleep, where you dream, where you make love. If you do it, try to break the habit. We've previously discussed some of the causes and remedies for excessive gaseousness [see chapter 6]. If they don't work for you, consult your doctor. He or she might help."

Appearance

Zinney continued, "Another thing for some of you guys and gals—we don't need to hide our age, but we sure don't have to advertise it either. Wearing clothes with food spots, and possibly even urine spots, suggests you don't care about personal hygiene. If you're dirty on the outside it seems reasonable to some people that you're probably dirty down under, that you have dirty socks and underwear and that your body is dirty. That's not aging gracefully. This slovenly appearance diminishes your dignity. It projects a lack of self-esteem. There's no reason why you guys can't shave or have a neatly-trimmed beard and have your hair trimmed and nicely combed.

"Also, some of you gals don't see as well as you used to. This is evident by the way some ladies apply make-up, like war masks. Sometimes it's so thick that it drips onto the collar of their blouses. At other times, it really looks like a mask. It stops at the chin instead of being blended lower. Get a better magnifying mirror, apply a little less perfume and make-up, and blend it in more smoothly. And *never ever* use these things as a substitute for cleanliness.

"You deserve to look like you care about yourself. If we don't care about ourselves, others won't really care either. This is all part of aging gracefully.

Positions for better sex

"To complete our discussion on this subject, let's say a few words about the sex act itself. Now I know I'm in a room full of experts here. And I hope that no one views this discussion as a porno class or excerpts from a sex manual. But I think this stuff is important. So, at the risk of being presumptuous, let me tell you about some positions that will help us as older adults enjoy intercourse a little more.

"The 'missionary position' is one that everybody understands. It's best described as the woman on the bottom and the man on top with the female partner's legs spread and the legs of the male partner between them [fig. 14E]. Listen to this simple variation of this position. After insertion of the penis into the vagina, the female part-

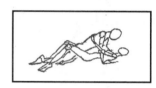

Fig 14E

ner slowly brings her legs inside the legs of her male partner.

"This position might prove to be a more comfortable for some partners, especially those with hip problems, or just an enjoyable variation for others.

"Many people, and this is somewhat more common among females, suffer from chronic abdominal discomfort. Sometimes this is the result of pelvic surgery and the development of adhesions, like from a hysterectomy or appendectomy. Sometimes it's due to chronic constipation or excessive gaseousness. You men have to think about the little ladies who have a sore belly. Imagine the terror they might experience when one of you big guys is about to jump on their sore belly.

"A reversal of the missionary position with the female partner on top [fig. 14F] can be particularly useful for couples when the male partner has low back problems or the female partner has abdominal problems.

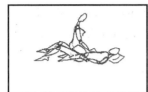

Fig 14F

"Another variation for men with low back discomfort is the 'sitting in the chair position.' In this situation, the male partner sits in a chair and the female straddles his thighs [fig. 14G].

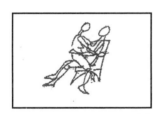

Fig 14G

"Still another position that might ameliorate or decrease a girl's abdominal discomfort during intercourse is the so-called *stallion on the mare* position. This is where the female partner is on her knees and her hands or on her elbows and knees, and the male partner assumes a position behind her [fig. 14H].

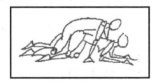
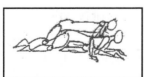

Fig 14H

"She can get some additional support by stacking two or three pillows beneath her lower abdomen and pelvis. The man partner is then able to insert his penis into the vagina from the rear, avoiding putting the pressure of his weight on the abdomen of the female partner.

"Now there are many other positions that might be of interest to you; but as I said, this is not meant to be a review of a sex manual. If you're interested in more, you can find one of those manuals in almost any bookstore."

Sam leaned over towards Craig and said, "I always called that last position 'doggie style.' This time, Craig, I have one for you. It's a story about John and Mary who were a very prim and proper couple about to celebrate their anniversary.

"John said to his wife, 'Honey, for our anniversary—let's do it doggie style.'

"She responded with fear and shock, 'No way! Why, I think that's crude and even borders on being disgusting.'

"'Aw, c'mon Mary,' pleaded John. 'It's really nothing of the kind. It'll be great—you'll like it.'

"'Well,' said Mary, 'I don't think so, but I will discuss it with our pastor before deciding on anything so drastic.' So Mary checked with her pastor, and to her amazement, he convinced her that there's nothing wrong between a husband and wife as long as it's consensual.

"Somewhat depressed, she returned to John. 'John, I checked with our pastor and he said it's ok to do it doggie style. So, I'll do it with you. But promise me, we'll only do it on a street where nobody knows us.'"

Oral sex

"I think it's important to say a few words about oral relationships, that is oral-genital relationships," Zinney continued. "Some of you view this negatively; but you would be surprised at how many folks really enjoy these pleasures. The important things here are twofold: cleanliness and consent. Good personal hygiene and cleanliness can make this activity pleasurable and poor personal hygiene can make it a real bad experience. Moreover, it's important that the activity be consensual. Forcing your partner or requiring your partner to indulge in an activity that he or she considers undesirable can be a real turn-off."

Sexually Transmitted Diseases [STDs]

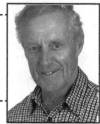

"What about sexually transmitted diseases?" asked Craig.

"Oral-genital relationships pose no additional hazard in this regard; but here again, cleanliness is an important preventative measure," said Zinney. "These diseases are less common in older adults because relationships are more likely to be monogamous. But make no mistake about it, older adults with multiple sexual partners are definitely at-risk. They should practice safe sex by using condoms and washing carefully.

"Now, are there any more questions? No? If there are no more questions, I'll see you next week. We'll take a phantom trip to the doctor's office; and while we're there, maybe we can get some advice on checkups and self-examination. Have a healthy week and I'll look forward to seeing you. By the way, that'll probably be our last session, so wear your party hat!"

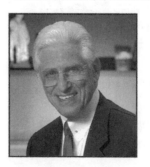

I'll make myself stronger,
I'll make love still longer!
I'll summon the gumption
For my share of consumption.

The Fountain of Age

The crowd milled into the auditorium knowing this was likely to be their last meeting. There was a festive feeling in the air that almost seemed like a high-school graduation party. Zinney appeared jubilant as he addressed the audience with a smiling welcome.

"Welcome to our last get-together. And let all of us view it as the start of your new beginning—the beginning of your second half. It's your 'tip off time.' During these past several weeks, all of you have learned a lot about aging. You've learned how to enhance the genetic influences of aging through nutrition and exercise—through physical and mental activity. This is what is meant by 'aging gracefully.'

"Many years ago the explorer Ponce de Leon searched deep in the jungles of Florida for the fabled 'Fountain of Youth.' During his journey, an arrow launched from the bow of a hostile Indian fatally pierced his heart. He was only forty-seven years old." Jokingly, Zinney continued, "He should have listened to his mother who sternly warned him. 'Poncey—better you should go to Philadelphia and look for the Fountain of Age than to go on a wild goose chase in the woods for the youth fountain.' Another example of mother knows best.

"So, what does aging gracefully actually mean? To some, it means passively and pleasantly accepting the disabilities of advancing age. But we've learned differently over these past few weeks. It is important to be active rather than passive. It is in this way that you can compress morbidity. As we've previously discussed, compression of morbidity is the true definition of aging gracefully. And again, what does that mean? What does compression of morbidity mean? It means staying healthy and independent for as long as possible, so that you may enjoy partaking in all of the magnificent wonders of life.

"To this end, no discussion or series of discussions on the subject of aging would be complete without addressing some of the medical aspects of maintaining good health. You should know what you should get checked, what you should check yourself, what screening tests you should have, and what vaccinations you should get to maintain good health.

An ounce of prevention

"It's much easier to prevent some diseases than to cure them. Some diseases can be effectively prevented by vaccinations; we'll discuss some of them a little later. Others diseases can be more effectively cured when identified in their early stages. How can we accomplish this? Well, the two most important ways to achieve early detection are first, self-awareness or self-examination, and second, periodic health screening examinations. You and your doctor should decide the best schedule for screening exams for

you. Both of you should thoroughly discuss issues relating to your health status, your age, and the history of any diseases in your family that could affect your future. These might include hereditary diseases or hereditary tendencies to develop certain problems such as heart disease, diabetes, colorectal cancer, breast cancer, and many others.

Self-examination of the genitals

"Let's discuss self-examination and awareness as the first order of business. All of you should examine your genital areas. Women should check for lumps, sores, warts, or any abnormal vaginal discharge. All of these are warning signs that should signal the need to seek medical advice.

"You boys should take note also. Cancer of the penis can be easily diagnosed in its early stages by self-exams. The same is true of testicular tumors. Testicular tumors are not as common in older men as they are in younger men and not nearly as common as breast cancer in women; but they do occur and can be diagnosed at an early stage by self-exam. So, check you penis and carefully examine each testicle. If you feel any lumps or any increase in size, see your doctor.

Self-examination of the breasts

"Ladies first. Ladies, please, please examine your own breasts. You can't rely on mammograms and doctor visits as the only source of detecting a lump. I can't tell you how many times I've seen patients with lumps in their breasts that proved to be cancer—cancer that did not show up on mammography. Mammograms are not foolproof. Although it is uncommon, men can also get breast cancer. So examine your little boobs following the same instructions that I give the ladies. I can understand that many people play the *ostrich* until they go to the doctor. But you can't do that. You can't be the ostrich. The stakes are too high and the results of early detection and treatment of breast cancer are too good. You can't allow a preventable catastrophe to develop because of your fear of finding something—something that can be cured.

"When you visit the doctor, make sure he or she does a breast examination as opposed to just ordering a mammogram. Again, mammography is a very good test; but it's not foolproof. Ask your doctor to show you the preferred way of self-examination of your breasts. Since many of you here tonight are between doctor visits and I want you to start this right away, let me give you a few tips.

"First, look at your breasts and then look at them again in a mirror. Use a good mirror in a well-lit room and look at your breasts from different angles. Stand in front of the mirror with your hands behind your head, then with your hands on your hips and then while bending slightly forward so that your breasts hang freely. It's not uncommon for one breast to appear slightly larger than the other; but see if you can detect any lumps, any retraction or inversion of the nipple, any skin changes at all, or any difference in the motion between the two breasts.

"Next, feel your breasts [fig. 15A]. Get used to the way your breasts feel so that if changes develop, you can detect them. It's a good idea to feel your breasts in two positions: lying down and also standing up. This is easy to do while showering. Don't use your fingertips; use the flat part of the ends of your fingers. The skin on the undersurface of the ends of your fingers is much

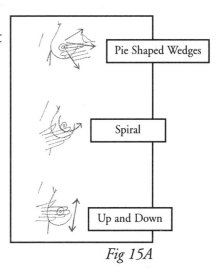

Fig 15A

259

more sensitive than the very tips. It may prove fruitful to use a little lubricant, moisturizing lotion, or soap and water while doing the exam. This will decrease the friction of your fingers against the skin of your breasts and increase your ability to detect changes.

"Divide the breast into four quadrants: the upper-outer, the upper-inner, the lower outer, and the lower-inner quadrants. Examine each quadrant of both breasts thoroughly and systematically. Use gentle pressure in small circular, searching movements.

"Examine your left breast with your right hand while your left hand is raised behind your head. Then, reverse the position of your hands to examine your right breast.

"Also, be sure to check deep in each armpit, or axilla, for lumps. To do this, put your fingers in your axilla and then lower your arm. This takes the tension off the muscles of the armpit. With your fingers now deeply placed in your axilla, repeat the same gentle circular examination.

"Then, carefully check each nipple for skin changes and gently squeeze each nipple between your thumb and index finger and check for a discharge. A cloudy discharge from squeezing the nipple is usually normal, but if it's bloody or brown, see your doctor.

"Suppose you feel something? Well, first of all, know that most lumps are not cancerous. They can be cysts or benign tumors or, on the other hand, they can be cancers. So if you find a lump or anything that puzzles you, get a professional opinion. Another thing, if you feel a lump and it's tender, that doesn't mean it isn't important. Usually, cancers are not tender; but they can be.

"Clumps of lumps can be the norm for many women. In fact, most women have some lumpiness and areas of thickness in their breasts. If it's the same on both sides, it's probably not significant. Check with your doctor if you note any of the following: your findings are not the same on each side, you feel something that's a departure from that which you usually feel, or you feel an area that is harder than the rest of your breast. For those of you who are still menstruating, it's a good idea to do your examinations a few days after your menstrual period when your breasts have returned to normal and are less engorged and swollen.

Mammograms

"Mammograms are special x-rays of the breast with the ability to detect tumors that are too small to feel. But as I said earlier, they're not foolproof.

Mammography should not be viewed as a substitute for having clinical exams by your physician or for performing regular self-examinations. Mammograms should be an addition to them. Also, if you know you have a lump, please tell the doctor. In such cases, the mammogram should be coupled with an ultrasound examination of the suspicious area.

"Many authorities recommend starting yearly mammograms at age fifty. In my opinion, they are best started at age forty; and, if not done yearly, then at least once every two years until age fifty. At fifty years of age, I think mammograms should be done every year. On the other hand, if a close relative, like your mother or sister, developed breast cancer in her thirties or forties, consider starting your mammograms and doctor examinations earlier. Please, ladies, please discuss this with your doctor.

Cervical cancer screening and pelvic examinations

"As you know, a pelvic examination consists of an internal vaginal examination by your doctor. In addition to visually inspecting your external genitalia, the doctor will do a bi-manual examination with two fingers of one hand in the vagina and with the other hand on the lower abdomen. In this way, he or she can search for abnormalities involving the uterus and ovaries.

"Following this, the doctor will insert a speculum into the vagina to visually evaluate the vagina and cervix of the uterus. At this time, a Pap smear test for cancer of the cervix can be performed. It's recommended that a Pap test be done every one to three years. The proper frequency of these examinations for you can best be determined in consultation with your doctor. For example, if you have significant risk factors, such as a history of genital warts or a family history of cervical cancer, it might be more appropriate for you to have the test annually. If, on the other hand, you have no risk factors, or if you've had a hysterectomy for reasons other than uterine or cervical cancer, you may not need annual exams.

Prostate cancer screening

"Prostate cancer is one of the more common causes of death in older men; and it's usually curable when detected and treated in the early stages. In some cases, there appears to be a family predisposition to it. It also seems more common in men who eat a high-fat diet and men of African-American descent. Most often it develops after the age of sixty-five, but it can occur earlier. In my opinion, initial screening should begin between the ages of forty-five to fifty.

"Prostate cancer screening is done by digital rectal examination and by a blood test known as the PSA. These letters stand for Prostatic Specific Antigen. This substance circulates in the blood in two forms. One is bound to a protein and the other is free or unbound. Sometimes, equivocal results in the total PSA can be clarified by determining the ratio of free PSA to bound PSA. Free PSA should be 20 percent or more of the total PSA. No test is foolproof, so have both the digital rectal exam and the blood test done every year. If an abnormality is detected, your doctor may want to do a biopsy. This is done through the rectum with the use of an ultrasound device that permits the targeting of several punch biopsies. But don't get frightened, boys. The procedure is a little uncomfortable, but not really painful.

"Of note is the fact that prostate cancer appears to be less dangerous in older aged men. Here it often grows more slowly and may not significantly affect longevity. It's more serious when contracted between the late forties and the early seventies, and appears to gradually decrease in virulence with advancing age. Because of this, many authorities question the value of the routine screening of the older gentlemen of our population.

"What additional health checkups and vaccinations should you expect from your doctor? A lot of this will depend on your age, on your risk factors, and the state of your health. Let's discuss some of these other issues with our focus directed to those things that would most benefit mature and older adults.

Blood pressure

"High blood pressure, also known as hypertension, is a real killer. It's associated with a high incidence of strokes, heart attacks, and congestive heart failure. Contrary to popular belief, it's not usually symptomatic. Most people with high blood pressure don't even know they have it. They don't have headaches or dizziness or any symptoms at all. Instead, this disease quietly progresses, like a thief in the night, to produce its evil effects. That's why you *must* have your blood pressure checked.

"If it is elevated, you should discuss the treatment options with your doctor. Sometimes the treatment is quite simple. It may only involve lifestyle modifications such as weight reduction, salt restriction, and exercise. At other times, medication is required.

If you have it, the first important step is to know you have it. So get your pressure checked. If it's elevated, get it taken care of and keep a careful watch on it.

"If there's a history of hypertension, strokes, or heart disease in your family or if you are African American, the risk of developing high blood pressure is greater; you're at high risk. While everyone should have his or her pressure checked at least once a year, if you're at high risk or if you know you have high pressure, the frequency of your pressure checks assumes even greater importance. This should be decided upon in consultation with your doctor. Relatively inexpensive and convenient home blood pressure machines can allow those of you in these situations to monitor your blood pressure at frequent intervals. This information can be of great value to the decision-making process you share with your physician.

Vision Evaluation

"The older we get, the less we see and hear. You've got to get your eyes and ears checked regularly. First, let's talk about some of the more common difficulties we experience with our eyes; and then we'll talk a little about hearing loss.

Presbyopia

"Needless to say, your sight is one of your most precious assets. Regardless of the cause, visual disturbances can affect your ability to balance, to walk, to negotiate stairs, and to avoid falls. All of us realize that our visual acuity changes as we get older. For the most part, vision can be corrected. As we age, the lens becomes less pliable and less able to change its shape to accommodate for seeing near objects. This part of the aging process is given the fancy name of *presbyopia*. While this change in our eyes actually begins in our teens, we usually don't require corrective lenses until we're forty years old or older. If you are beginning to have difficulty reading the fine print, get your vision checked. A good pair of spectacles can make a world of difference and save you a lot of grief.

Cataracts

"Cataracts are opacities that develop in the lens [fig. 15B]. These opacities

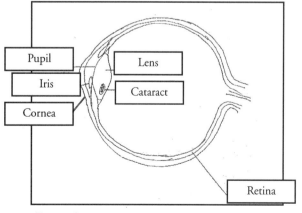

Fig 15B

263

cloud the clarity of the lens in a manner similar to fog or a spot on the lens of your eyeglasses. While there are many factors that contribute to the development of cataracts, they are commonly the consequence of degenerative changes that occur with aging. These opacities can cause a progressive and painless loss of vision. Frequent changes in eyeglass prescriptions can often maintain useful vision. When this fails, surgery can usually be expected to produce excellent results.

Glaucoma

"Glaucoma is a condition characterized by an increase in the pressure within the eyeball. It usually comes on gradually, but can develop suddenly. It can cause anything from slightly impaired vision to complete blindness. Symptoms, such as seeing a halo around lights, pain, pressure in an eye, headaches, and vague visual disturbances, should sound an alert. Those who are at greatest risk are people older than the age of thirty-five years, those with a family history of glaucoma, and patients with diabetes. While there are different types of glaucoma and many causes for the condition, it is usually an easy diagnosis for your ophthalmologist to make. More encouraging, the majority of cases can be adequately treated with medicine or surgery.

Macular degeneration

"A more troublesome condition is macular degeneration. Macular degeneration is the leading cause of serious visual impairment in the elderly. It produces a progressive loss of central vision; and while the onset is usually gradual, sometimes it's catastrophically sudden. Although there is no adequate medical treatment, laser therapy is occasionally helpful in cases that are identified early. Intensive research is underway to find a cure or a method of prevention. Hopefully, a breakthrough is not far away.

Diabetic retinopathy

"Diabetic retinopathy causes a deterioration of the retina. It's a major cause of blindness in diabetics and is worsened by hypertension. Good control of diabetes and blood pressure is important in retarding the development of this problem; but unfortunately, it won't reverse it after it's been established. Fortunately, laser therapy can produce improvement in some cases when identified early.

Laser surgery

"The correction of visual problems with the use of laser therapy, and more recently radiotherapy, has received wide public attention. Surgical techniques using laser treatments have allowed many to abandon their spectacles. The procedure is quick, relatively painless, and is associated with a low incidence of complications. While this form of treatment has not yet proven effective in presbyopia, further improvement in equipment and refinement in techniques are anticipated. Still investigational, radiotherapy has recently been used to change the convexity of the cornea, enabling some to read without glasses. Both laser treatment and radiotherapy are likely to be particularly appealing to those who disdain the use of eyeglasses. However, their long-term benefits have not yet been completely evaluated and we look forward to the results of these studies with great hope.

"I've only just touched on the myriad of problems that can affect your eyes. However in light of what we've discussed, I'm sure that all of us can appreciate the importance of regular vision checkups and eye examinations. So schedule them with your doctor. In particular, diabetic patients should have their eyes checked at least once a year by an ophthalmologist. These examinations should include a visual acuity evaluation, eye pressure measurements, and a thorough examination of the retina. But should any of you develop visual difficulty, eye pain, or eye pressure between your sched-uled routine examinations, seek medical advice as soon as possible. Now, let's talk a little about your ears.

Hearing

"There is a host of diseases that can cause hearing loss. Many of these can be successfully treated—a good reason to get your hearing checked if you think you're a victim. However, our main interest here is to discuss the common form of hearing loss associated with aging. Its medical name is *presbycusis*, but you don't have to remember the scientific terminology. This condition causes progressive hearing loss as we get older. Actually, it can begin as early as age twenty as a result of stiffening and deterioration of some structures of the inner ear. Some of us may become severely impaired by the time we're sixty, while others seem relatively unaffected even into our nineties. The degree of impairment is extremely variable."

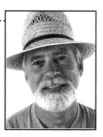

"Doc, John Kinder here. Do you think exposure to loud noises has anything to do with this condition?"

"Yes, I do," Zinney answered. "People who have prolonged exposure to loud noise in the workplace or who expose themselves to it by habitually listening

265

to loud music seem more likely to develop it earlier and possibly even more severely. This may be one of the reasons it's more common in men. However, the more interesting thing about this condition is the failure of the victim to recognize it in its early stages. This is either because its slowly progressive or very often because of denial—you know, 'I'm not hard of hearing, not me.' Commonly, relatives or friends first notice the situation and when they mention it to the afflicted, it's firmly denied or casually dismissed.

"For the many of us who suffer from this, let's all appreciate that it's a common consequence of aging. It's nothing to be ashamed of. But not doing something about it may become something to be ashamed of, because you're missing a lot. There are parts of conversations you're not getting or not understanding—because you didn't hear them correctly or because you didn't hear enough of it to understand. You might misinterpret parts of a conversation and then make a comment that's totally out of context. If your colleagues don't recognize your problem, it's likely that they'll think you're less intelligent than you really are. They're likely to think you're losing it a little, or worse, that you're a doddering old fool that can be easily deceived.

"More importantly, the input to your knowledge base is decreased. If you don't hear what you're supposed to hear, you won't know some of the things you should know. You will be less knowledgeable than you should be. You'll be less valuable than you could be. But you're not an old fool; you're not demented; you just can't hear.

"So, what should you do if your loved ones tell you they think you're having a hearing problem? First, you should thank them. Then, for God's sake, get your ears and hearing checked! You might be a good candidate for a hearing aid. Many of these newer devices are small, comfortable, more effective, and more easily concealed than the older versions. And if you need a larger version, so what?! Don't let ego stand in the way of your awareness or of your ability to learn new information. Even more promising is the development of a device that can be surgically implanted. While still in the developmental stage, it holds great promise for the future."

"It seems as we get older the number of problems we face just keep increasing and increasing with no end in sight," Craig whispered to Sam.

"Well," Sam replied, "you have to keep it in perspective and you can't lose your sense of humor. It reminds me of this ninety-five year old man with thick eyeglasses and large hearing aids in each ear who was wandering the streets of Manhattan. As he got more and more confused, he walked into St. Patrick's Cathedral and directly into a confessional booth.

"The priest on the other side of the partition said, 'Tell me, my son, how can I help you?' The old man heard nothing and so he didn't reply. The priest repeated this several times and after getting no reply became frustrated and knocked on the partition, to which the old man responded, 'Listen, buddy. You can stop with the knocking and the banging. There's no paper in this booth either.'"

Tinnitus

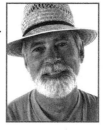

"That's great information, Doc," said John. "I think I understand that presby-whatcha-call-it hearing problem. But you know, a lot of us have trouble with ringing in our ears. I know I do. Sometimes it drives me crazy, especially at night. Do we grow bells or buzzers in our ears when we get older or what? Every time I go to the doctor and tell him about it he poo-poos it. What's that all about?"

"You've touched on a very common problem," said Zinney. "It's called *tinnitus*, and it comes in many different costumes. It can be a ringing, a hiss-ing, a roaring, or a buzzing. It may be constant or intermittent and most people find it particularly annoying at night—when they're lying in bed. This is probably because it's quiet and the sounds of the day don't block it out. The actual cause of tinnitus is obscure. Most of the time it's benign—it's not related to a serious condition. What we do know is that it can be associated with almost any disorder of the ear, nose, or throat or even disturbances in other systems, like the cardiovascular system. Heavy tobacco use and even some medications, like aspirin, have been blamed. Also, it's commonly associated with some degree of hearing loss. So anyone with tinnitus should have their hearing checked and have a thorough examination of their ears, nose, and throat. The doctor may recommend additional testing in some instances, but the condition should not, as you say, be 'poo-pooed.'

"The reason some doctors make light of the situation is sometimes both good news and bad news. The good news is that your physician may have already satisfied himself that you have the common form of benign tinnitus. There is no identifiable cause for this common type, and there are no serious diseases associated with it. That's the good news.

"The bad news is that there is no known cure. Rest, avoidance of stress, cessation of smoking, medication changes, and the like, have all met with varying degrees of success. Sometimes sound-blocking devices can be beneficial. However, like in any other medical situation, if you feel you're getting short shrift in regard to your complaints, get another opinion.

Colorectal cancer screening

"Moving on, colon cancer is one of the more common killers in our society. Most of these cancers begin as benign polyps (benign growths) that can be removed through a colonoscope. When cancer does develop, the cure rates from surgery are very good—providing a diagnosis is made early. Early diagnosis and cure can be achieved through screening tests. These screening tests involve checking the stool for the presence of blood, examining the colon with x-ray studies, and examining the colon by direct visualization with the use of flexible instruments.

Fecal occult blood test

"Most experts recommend that your stool be tested for the presence of blood once a year after the age of fifty. This test is called an FOBT. It stands for Fecal Occult Blood Test. Having a positive test doesn't necessarily mean you have cancer or a polyp; and having a negative test doesn't mean that you don't have one. But it appears to be a useful screening test in identifying patients at high risk and encouraging further evaluation.

Flexible sigmoidoscopy and colonoscopy

"Also, most experts recommend a flexible sigmoidoscopy after the age of fifty. But they disagree on how frequently they should be performed after that. Opinions range from every three to every ten years. These differences in opinion have yet to be resolved but they don't apply to people in a high risk category. Individuals with a family history of colon cancer or colon polyps in a first or second degree relative and those who have colon disorders, like ulcerative colitis, are examples of patients at high risk. Most would agree that individuals who are at high risk for developing colon cancer should have a complete colonoscopy, not just a flexible sigmoidoscopy, about every three to five years.

"Moreover, if your father, mother, or a sibling developed colon cancer, you should probably start your checkups ten years before the diagnosis was made in them. So you see, the age at which you start your checkups and the type of evaluations that should be performed is often related to your individual risk factors."

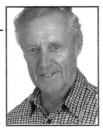

"That's good to know, Doc," said Craig. "But I'm a little confused between a sigmoidoscopy and a colonoscopy."

Flexible sigmoidoscopy

"I should have explained that," Zinney said. "A lot of people don't know the difference. A flexible sigmoidoscopy is a shorter examination that checks the lower part of your colon and your rectum. The instrument is inserted into the rectum and advanced into the lower colon, or the sigmoid colon. The length of the instrument is usually sixty-five centimeters, so it can be used to examine about twenty-five inches of the lower colon and the rectum. The examination is a little uncomfortable, but not usually painful. In selected instances, your doctor might recommend a lower GI x-ray study (barium enema) to examine the rest of your colon.

Colonoscopy

"A colonoscopy examines the entire colon. This examination requires more extensive preparation, in the form of laxatives and a day or two of dietary restrictions. It's usually done with the use of sedation and pain medication."

"I should hope so," said Craig. "That sounds like a major Owee."

"Yeah," Sam added. "It sounds like a Giant Goose. You should give that test the Latin name of Goosus-Maximus."

"This could be a useful psychological examination for some people," chuckled Craig. "We might find out where they keep their brains and what their brains are made of." Then as he struggled to control himself he added, "Just kidding."

"Now, now, boys," Zinney commented. "Because of the excellent sedation that's usually used for colonoscopy, the procedure is rarely painful. Most people don't even remember it after it's over. The most difficult part of the whole thing is the preparation, and that's not all that bad. Many of my patients have told me this.

Virtual colonoscopy

"And there is a more promising development on the horizon called 'virtual colonoscopy.' This is a test that examines the colon with a special CT x-ray, a cat scan, which can be performed painlessly and quickly. While the technique is still undergoing study and improvement, it seems likely to become a cost-effective, painless, and convenient way to screen most people for colon tumors in the not-too-distant future."

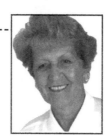

"I've been told that after the age of eighty, there's no good reason to do colon screening tests. How do you feel about that?" asked Miriam.

"I've heard that opinion expressed many times but I couldn't disagree more," Zinney replied. "If you're going to do something about a disease when you diagnose it, then you should do screening tests for it. The decision to screen or not to screen should always be individualized.

"We'll talk more about this controversy a little later, but a good example of this is a patient of mine named Marjorie. Although she didn't know her family history at the time of her own ordeal, we later found that her mother died of colon cancer at the age of eighty-three. Even later, it was determined that her aunt also succumbed to colon cancer at the age of eighty-five. Marjorie was luckier, because we found her colon cancer at the age of eighty-two by doing a routine screening test for blood in the stool. This test was positive and led to

a colonoscopy. The colonoscopy identified the cancer and led to a successful surgical cure. Fourteen years later, Marjorie is now ninety-six years old and still living independently in her own apartment.

Cholesterol and blood sugar determinations

"We've previously discussed the importance of your blood cholesterol and the desirable range for total cholesterol and for HDL and LDL [see chapter 6]. But when should you start to have these checked? Most authorities feel that men should start cholesterol screening at thirty-five years of age and continue it through age sixty-five or longer. Women should do the same starting at forty-five years of age.

"You may have one of many risk factors that indicate the need for you to have your cholesterol checked more frequently. To mention a few high-risk conditions: a family history of early heart attack, a history of tobacco use, elevated cholesterol, diabetes, or high blood pressure. Your risk factors need to be clearly identified and discussed with your physician. The same is true for your blood sugar. Anyone can get diabetes and you're at greater risk if you have a family history of diabetes, if you're overweight, or if you eat a lot of sugar. So, get your sugar checked.

270

Flu and pneumonia vaccinations

"Now, let's talk a little about vaccination as it applies to us older folks. Older adults and particularly those with chronic pulmonary or cardiac conditions are very susceptible to the complications of the flu and pneumonia. The Center for Disease Control (CDC) has done a wonderful job in predicting the particular strain of flu viruses that are most likely to hit us each year. They have missed from time to time, but they're getting better and better at it. Based on their predictions, a new flu vaccine that usually protects against three different viruses, is produced each year.

"That's why it is sometimes in short supply. It takes several weeks to develop immunity after receiving the vaccine but the immunity lasts for about six months. I highly recommend that older adults take this shot every year unless their doctor suggests otherwise. He or she may recommend against it because of a history of adverse reactions or an allergy that you might have.

"Pneumonia vaccinations are available for a particular kind of pneumonia known as pneumococcal pneumonia—not for all kinds of pneumonia. Among older adults, pneumococcal pneumonia is responsible for numer-ous deaths each year. The vaccination used to be recommended as a once-in-a-lifetime shot; but now, most authorities suggest it be repeated every five years. You should take this shot and save yourself the grief of a very serious illness.

Controversy over preventative health screening in the elderly

"Finally, there's a great deal of controversy as to the efficacy of cholesterol and cancer screening in older age groups. In fact, preventative health-screening tests and periodic physical examinations, in general, have come under scrutiny—particularly in the elderly. In the minds of some authorities, the costs and the disparity between supply and demand have indicated the need for rationing medical services—even some vaccines. They have pointed to the lack of statistical benefit expected from some screening tests as a reason to restrict them to younger people. For example, statistics demonstrate that the average 75 year old woman will most likely live another twelve years and that giving up Pap smears would result in an average loss of only three days of life expectancy. Also, giving up mammograms and fecal occult blood tests would be at a statistical cost of only nine days of longevity.

"Even abandoning the routine use of mammograms at the early age of fifty only seems to cost forty-three days of longevity—a difference of a little more than one month. Do these statistically-derived findings favor doing these screening tests? Not on the face of it. But that's not what health-screening tests are about. These are averages. They're not applicable to individuals like 96-year-old Marjorie who had her colon cancer diagnosed and successfully treated at the age of eighty-two, all because of a screening test.

"Health screening tests are performed to find those individuals who can benefit from early diagnosis and treatment. Clearly, it makes no sense to screen for diseases that are not likely to occur in the older age groups, like chlamydia and gonorrhea. And it also makes no sense to screen for a disease where the treatment poses a greater threat to the individual than the disease itself. The question we must always ask is whether or not the benefits outweigh the hazards of diagnosis and treatment for a given condition in a given individual. If the answer to that question is yes, and there is a simple screening test for that disease, then the test should be made available to that individual. To do otherwise, to apply statistical averages to an individual, will imbed age discrimination into health care policy.

"What is really important is the health status of the individual. A determination must be made for each individual as to whether or not the treatment of a commonly-encountered disease would benefit that individual, based on their projected longevity. Some in the health care community may think that's too hard to do—it's easier to establish arbitrary age limits for cancer and cholesterol screening. Too bad! That's our job! If a 75-year-old individual has a projected life expectancy of twenty years instead of the average twelve years, then surely he or she should have selected screening tests. On the other hand, if a less healthy 55 year old individual has a life expectancy of only two or three years, perhaps certain screening tests can be foregone.

"Add to all of this the likelihood of further increasing functional longevity. Might we not find a cure for Alzheimer's disease during the next ten years? Moreover, falls are among the major causes of death above the age of eighty-five. Can we not decrease the frequency of falls, perhaps by 50 percent, through strength and balance training programs? Might we not discover newer and better anti-aging treatments through investigating the human genome? These are real possibilities—not 'pie in the sky' goals. When one realizes how dramatically these changes could alter the equation, the need for prevention of disease and screening tests in older adults enters a new dimension. Recognizing this, the possibility of age discrimination improperly insinuating itself into our health care system must be diligently avoided. All of us must be cautiously aware of how a well-meaning scientific community's statistical efforts can be improperly used by a sometimes not-so-well meaning bureaucracy. Statistics can sometimes be likened to a drunk leaning on a lamppost: *used more for support than enlightenment.*

"Well, I did blow off a lot of steam tonight! It's getting to be that time again—time to say goodnight and join some of you night owls in the back of the room for refreshments. I must say these last several weeks have been a joy for me. It's been a pleasure working with you and getting to know you. I'll miss each and every one of you; and I do hope our paths cross again. In the meantime, please remember, we can WIN. Each and every one of us can WIN in the second half. You may feel the pain of getting old or the pain derived from others implying you're too old. Don't be disheartened. As they say in the world of sports when things are not quite as good as they could be, suck it up. So, suck it up, my friends, and forge

ahead. You may have to collect your fortitude, but you can do it.

"A friend of mine wrote a poem called 'The Great Rewind.' I think it sums it up for all of us. Last week I asked a small group of you to learn the different parts of this poem and participate in its recitation tonight. I'll start it off and we'll finish the last four lines together."

The Great Rewind

"In ways, I am told,
I'm getting too old,
That my brain is too dim
And my thoughts are too grim.

While I'm certain to die
When my years have passed by,
I still pray that my Keeper
Will stay the Grim Reaper.

But the Reaper's distraction
Depends on my action,
And the choices I make
To secure my stake.

So I'll summon the gumption
To control my consumption,
And make myself stronger
To keep fit yet longer.

I'll gather the grit
To sharpen and restore my wit
And harvest the hustle
To strengthen and rebuild my muscle.

(All together)

Then, when my strength does rewind
And, as well, my mind,
I will clearly behold
That the rest can be gold."

"Splendid, splendid folks," Zinney exclaimed. "Now my good friends, now the second half begins—the second half of the game of life. You could even view it as a race, the length of which will be different for each of us. It might be a year for some or more than fifty years for others. But unlike any other race, those of us that cross the finish line with fuel in our tanks and air still in our tires, are the real winners. This is our understanding of compressing morbidity or aging gracefully. This is your Fountain of Age. So please, ladies and gentlemen—Start Your Engines and enjoy the ride."

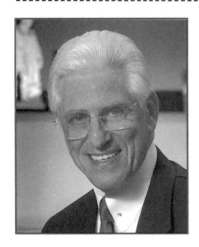

NOTES

284